Religion, Spirituality and Healthcare

Other Books from the Author

The Invisible Temple, Llewellyn 1987.
Apocalypse Now, Llewellyn 1988.
Divine Light and Fire, Element Books, 1992 (reprint, Vega, 2002).
Divine Light and Love, Element Books, 1994 (reprint, Vega, 2002).
The Sociological Adventure, Kendall-Hunt, 1996.
Prayer: The Royal Path of the Spiritual Tradition, Xlibris, 2003.
Medicine and Spirituality: The Encounter of the 21ˢᵗ Century, Xlibris, 2004.
What are Life and Death on Earth? Xlibris, 2004.
What are Wisdom and Scientific Knowledge? Xlibris, 2004.
The Spiritual Family in the 21ˢᵗ Xlibris, 2005.
Essential Encounters, Vol. I (2006), Vol. II (2007), Easy Stroudsburg University Publ.

In French

L'Alternance Instinctive (with Jacques Pezé), Louise Courteau, Ed. 1993.
La Voie Initiatique de l'An 2000, Louise Courteau, Ed. 1994.
Les Vitamines d'Amour, Editions de l'Aigle, 1998.
L'Homme Gratte-ciel, Editions de l'Aigle, 2002.
Les Fleurs de la Vie, Vol. I, II, III, IV, Le Dauphin Blanc, 2001-2003.
La Prière, Le Dauphin Blanc, 2003.
Médecine et Spiritualité: Le grand Rendez-vous du XXIe Siècle, Le Dauphin Blanc, 2004
La Famille Spirituelle au 21ᵉ Siècle, Le Dauphin Blanc, 2005.

In Italian

Lo Sviluppo dell'Uomo Nuovo, Vol. I, II, III, Eta' dell'Acquario 1989-1991.
I livelli della Coscienza, Eta' dell'Acquario 1997.
Luce e Fuoco Divino, IDM, 1998.
Amore e Luce Divina, IDM, 1998.
Iniziazione al terzo Millennio, IDM, 1999.
L'Amore, come capirlo e viverlo, Elvetica Edizioni, 2002.
Le Vitamine d'Amore, IDM, 2003
La Salute Globale, Elvetica Edizioni, 2003
Medicina e Spiritualita', Guna, 2003.
La Preghiera: Strumento di Guarigione Olistica, Guna, 2004.
La Scintilla Divina: Il piu' grande Mistero e Tesoro, Guna, 2004.
Il Perdono: Strumento essenziale di Guarigione e Benessere, Guna, 2004.
Il Destino: Perche' siamo quello che siamo e viviamo quell,o che viviamo?, Guna, 2005.
Il Pellegrinaggio: Risveglio alla Realta', Guna, 2006.
Incontro con Santi e Saggi, Guna, 2006.
La Famiglia Spirituale, Anima, 2006.
Medicina Differenziale e Qualitativa, Guna 2007.
La Natura Umana: lo Sforzo e la Grazia, Guna, 2007.

Religion, Spirituality and Healthcare

How to Understand Them
and Live Them Today

Peter Roche de Coppens, Ph.D.

Library of Congress Control Number:		2007902474
ISBN:	Hardcover	978-1-4257-6889-8
	Softcover	978-1-4257-6884-3

To order additional copies of this book, contact:
Xlibris Corporation
1-888-795-4274
www.Xlibris.com
Orders@Xlibris.com
30036

Contents

INTRODUCTION 11

Part I: The Major World Religions

Introduction: The Beginning of the journey 21

Chapter I: What human beings really want, the answer of religion....................23

Chapter II: Hinduism 25

Chapter III: Confucianism 31

Chapter IV: Taoism..37

Chapter V: Buddhism..41

Chapter VI: Judaism..50

Chapter VII: Christianity 59

Chapter VIII: Islam 70

Conclusion and synopsis...79

Part II: Religion and Spirituality,
their relationship and distinctive characteristics

Introduction 91

Chapter I: Religion and Spirituality in the 21st century.....................................99

Chapter II: The Church, the image of human nature 120

Chapter III: The Christmas Story, the birth of spiritual consciousness................132

Chapter IV: The Easter Story, the archetype of Resurrection.............................143

Chapter V: Grace and spiritual energy 151

Chapter VI: Quintessential Christianity or the Ageless Wisdom.........................164

Chapter VII: The new Encyclopedia, A Compendium of Human Knowledge

                     for the 21st Century...173

Conclusion and synopsis...193

Part III: Religion and Spirituality: their role for healthcare, wellness, and the holistic medicine of the future

Introduction 201

Chapter I: The great challenges of our times, their dangers

                and opportunities 205

Chapter II: Essential presuppositions, intuitions,

                core insights and ideas..211

Chapter III: The role of religion and spirituality in medical practice 224

Chapter IV: Core contributions of religion and spirituality

                to the medical profession and healthcare in general........................234

Chapter V: How to integrate religion and spirituality

                in one's life and profession? 240

Conclusion...243

CONCLUSION...247

BIBLIOGRAPHY 253

Dedication

This work is dedicated with much love and appreciation to those who have combined a passion and dedication to authentic spirituality and effective healing on a truly integral basis . . . and to those who will follow in their foot steps. It is dedicated in particular to Maître Philippe de Lyons, Brother André and Bruno Groening, to Lydie Popineau, Mother Serena, and Gianna Pozzi. It is also dedicated to those medical doctors and healthcare specialists who are true "missionaries", who have come in this world to help the sick and suffering regardless of the efforts, sacrifices, and difficulties that were involved. Finally, it is dedicated to those who tirelessly are seeking to establish a "connection" between this side and the other side that, together, we may be more effective in understanding, sustaining and restoring health and holiness, Maguy Lebrun and Daniel Lemieux in particular.

"In India one must distinguish between religion and the personal spiritual life of each person. Religion constitutes a set of beliefs that bring with them a set of traditional rites, superstitions, and habits that culminate in a given life-style. Then comes spiritual life that frees itself from these obligations to find, through yoga, union with the supreme Reality, the essence of all things" (André Siegfried)

Introduction

As we cross over from the 20th to the 21st Century and enter into the third Millennium, a tremendous qualitative and quantitative transformation in taking place all over the world, both at the macro level of society and at the micro level of the individual. Human consciousness, the true "key" or explanatory instrument and process of human knowledge, is, unquestionably and inexorably shifting, transforming and expanding itself as we climb on our inner "sky-scraper" and rise on the "vertical axis of consciousness". Knowledge, sensibilities, priorities and energies are literally imploding and exploding. This, in turn, leads to a great deal of confusion, disorientation, and suffering; it leads to violence and thus insecurities and fears both in society and in the individual. As a result, the most important social institutions, the very "cradle" of both the individual and of society are all "crumbling" from within as scandals, corruption, vices, confusion and transformation rocks their very foundation.

It is no wonder, therefore, that the individual is confused, cut adrift on the "ocean of life" and desperately searching for something that makes sense, for meaningful answers, and valid "points of reference". Now one of the most important aspects of his life and being, as well as a truly fundamental social institution, has always been religion . . . and the spiritual dimension. Why? Because a human being has always been fundamentally a religious being (*homo religiosus*). The central theme and the focus of this new book will be *Religion, Spirituality and Healthcare*, underpinned by the truly essential questions, "can religion remain a vital and meaningful force in the 21st Century? How can the individual tap his human and spiritual resources and potential so as to live an authentic and fruitful spiritual life—how can he awaken and nourish his spiritual consciousness? Finally, how can he better understand and utilize religion and spirituality to preserve and restore his health and well-being—what impact can religion and spirituality have on the new paradigm of health and medicine emerging in the 21st century?

Underlying our essential theme and its primary focus are three axiological points, or fundamental premises, that will determine all the rest as well as the rationality and coherence of my presentation. These are:

1. A vision or conception of *human nature*: what is a human being?
2. A vision or conception of the *human psyche*: what is human consciousness, how does it unfold and how can we expand it?
3. A vision and conception of *human knowledge*: what constitutes human knowledge, how valid is it, and how do we obtain it and verify it?

These three axiological points are, clearly, a function of the level of consciousness and being—of evolution—of the person so that on different levels we get different conceptions as we do by raising or lowering our level of consciousness and being! Fundamentally, however, there are three basic positions that one can take, rationally and coherently. These are: a human being is a *homo simplex, duplex,* or *triplex;* that is, he has one essential nature, his physical body and its biochemical processes. Or he has two essential natures which are interrelated, the body (his biopsychic nature) and the psyche (his human or psychosocial nature made of emotions and thoughts which arise from, but become independent of, his physical body). Or he has three essential natures, the body, the psyche, and his soul and spiritual Self (his spiritual nature). This difference is truly fundamental and is the kingpin of all the assumptions and their derivatives that will follow.

If a human being is a *homo simplex*, if he is his biological organism and nothing else, then he is a biological machine that can best be understood in terms of mechanistic and organismic terms—of Newtonian physics; he comes from nothing and will return to nothing and there is no life and consciousness either before or after his biological death. His consciousness (cognitive processes, sensibilities, and will) are merely *epiphenomena* of biochemical processes. His senses (seeing and hearing in particular) and his reason (extended and expanded by various machines) are the best avenues for obtaining knowledge. He is determined by both internal and external physical factors and true free will is but an illusion, wishful thinking on his part. He is alone in the universe that is at best indifferent and the product of random chance and evolution. Material wealth and consumer goods are his essential wealth; competition is thus king in this world and egoism is the "iron law" of his life with power, material power, being the ultimate value and point of reference.

On the other hand, if a human being is a *homo duplex*, if he has a biological organism but also a human consciousness, or psyche, that emerges from his biological organism and that can acquire a life of its own and become a causal and creative factor, then he is more that a biological machine and needs to be understood in terms of both physical and psychological factors that, in turn are both internal and external. While he comes from nothing he may he evolve into something that will survive his biological death—that is his identity, consciousness and will may, somehow, survive. His consciousness is more than an epiphenomenon and may acquire an identity and level *sui generis* that may not be explained in a reductionistic fashion by material factors alone.

In addition to his senses and reason, he may also use his own personal experiences (phenomenology) and introspection as valid avenues for obtaining valid knowledge. Here, moreover, he may well be caught between two great and opposed forces, *determinism*, being bound by natural law, and *free will*, his ability to make choices. He may or may not be alone in the universe that may be indifferent or that may be benevolent to him and he may well be more than the product of random chance and evolution. His essential wealth may shift or fluctuate between material and psychic factors such as knowledge, love, and creativity; cooperation and altruism may also emerge in his consciousness while the ultimate value may also shift to justice, character and integrity—to a care for the common good.

Finally, if a human being is a *homo triplex*, if he has not only a biological organism, a human psyche but also a genuine spiritual nature then things change substantially. Life and consciousness, thus knowledge, love, and will—identity—may emerge not from matter alone but may, indeed, come from *elsewhere* to manifest in matter through psychic and material instruments. Here, he can best be understood in terms of modern, posteinsteinian and quantum physics as well as of transpersonal psychology and religion. He may also come from "elsewhere", from the spiritual worlds, to return to these spiritual worlds after the dissolution of his body so that life, consciousness, and identity may exist both *before* and *after* his birth and death. The true essence and origin of his nature may be spiritual rather than psychic or material and if this is so, then he may, indeed, be a microcosm of the macrocosm, a fractal of the ultimate reality where all levels and dimensions of reality intersect.

He may then, as Chinese philosophy and religion have always argued, be the "middle kingdom", the meeting point between heaven and earth, the physical and the spiritual, the outer and the inner, the male and female polarities, and all the opposites such as the very big and the very small, life and death, good and evil, etc. The avenues for obtaining knowledge are thus amplified to include intuition and inspiration in addition to the senses, reason, and personal experience. He may also be far from being alone in the universe and created by a much greater Intelligence and Power than his own for a definite plan and purpose; and the universe may be far from indifferent to him, it may be a "mirror" that sends back to him whatever he sends out into that universe! Here he is conditioned and governed by the laws and principles of each of the great planes of being that make up his being and the universe while retaining essential free will and the power of choice.

Thus, the truly fundamental question boils down to a very simple yet quite profound question with great many rational implications and practical applications: what is your conscious or unconscious, overt or covert, vision and conception of human nature—**what is man**? A *biological machine*, a *biological machine endowed with consciousness* that can then assume control of his destiny, or a *spiritual being* who is the synthesis of all there is and the intersection, or meeting, point of all dimensions and aspects, and potentialities of the universe? Directly related to the first question is the second axiological point: what is your vision or conception of the human psyche—**what is human consciousness**: its structure, functions, and manifestations? To answer that question I would direct you to Psychosynthesis and my work on the human psyche. Suffice it to say that here, too, we can have an essentially materialistically oriented vision, a psychosocially oriented vision or a spiritual vision with their ensuing implications and applications.

The third and final axiological point, which is very closely related and following the first two, is a vision or conception of human knowledge, **what is knowledge**, how valid is it, how do we obtain it and how do we verify it? Human knowledge can come from many sources and through different avenues. For most people and for science in particular it must be consensually validated and accepted and, unquestionably, it is a function of our level of consciousness and being. At the first level, knowledge is what I feel and experience, my inner realizations which are essentially sensory and instinctual. At the second level, it is based on our senses, reason, and human experience and must be repeatable so that if other people use the same procedures, they should obtain the same results. Finally, it can also be based on intuition and inspiration, which must then be validated through reason and the senses, and which finds its final expression and validation through our own *direct personal experience*.

At our present level of consciousness and being, the form of "knowledge" that is best known, validated by our collective level of consciousness and our core institutions, that enjoys the greatest acceptance and prestige, (namely scientific knowledge and academic knowledge) is the one based on the senses, reason, and that is consensually validated. Government, economics, politics, education, medicine and even religion have taken that "middle-range" type of knowledge as their fundamental "point of reference" and "yardstick"! It has taken us far but it has also cut out some of the knowledge that we obtained instinctually and through imitation of tradition and it has not yet reach the kind of knowledge that we can obtain through authentic intuition and inspiration and which must be personally experienced.

There is also a major difference in the way in which we can get intellectual, book-knowledge and lived, experiential knowledge. To get the first, we must attend a university, seminary or institute, pass their qualifying exams, and develop our reason and thinking powers but without putting our personal lives on the line. The second, on the other hand, is a direct result of what *we are* which is inextricably interconnected with how *we live*! This is why monasteries, retreats, spiritual elders, and a holistic frame of reference are truly essential for the second kind of knowledge. Here, you know what you are and how you live and not what you read, think about or discuss! The price to pay for experiential knowledge is much greater but so is also what it can do for you.

My fundamental answers to the questions: "What do human beings really want?" Can religion remain a vital and meaningful force in the 21st Century?" And "how can the individual tap his human and spiritual resources and potential so as to live an authentic and fruitful spiritual life?" are very simple and basic . . . yet *paradoxical*: Yes, if the esoteric aspects of religion are linked with the exoteric aspects, if the spirit can, once again, vivify the "letter" of religion and if the individual, each person (meaning **you**) will do the required work! And it is "No" if religion cannot undergo the basic changes in its interpretation and application of its symbols, rites, and parables which our present level of human consciousness and evolution are demanding, and if the individual refuses to do personal transformational work! Thus, the truly crucial question boils down to: how can we build a bridge between the esoteric and exoteric aspects of religion, relate religion to authentic spirituality, "vivify the letter with the spirit", and come up a new interpretation of the basic cosmic and eternal truths that religion channels? This is what constitutes the very essence of my work and its most basic thesis.

To answer that truly fundamental question we need to ask other questions such as: what is religion and what is it designed to do? What are the most important world religions? To what extent are these alike and to what extent are they different? What is spirituality and what can it do for us? What is the relationship between religion and spirituality? Finally (and most importantly), how can religion and spirituality help us to live in a more conscious, responsible, healthy, creative and joyful way? Last but not least, what role can religion and spirituality play for our healthcare in general and for the medicine of the future in particular? It is to answer these very basic questions that this book has been conceived. After due consideration, I decided to subdivide it into three basic parts: First, to give a brief synopsis of the four Eastern and three major Western world religions taking Huston Smith, a world renown authority as my basic frame of reference; second, to analyze the relationship between religion and spirituality; and third to relate religion and spirituality to wellness and a holistic medical approach of the future.

To answer these very important questions that touch the very core of our being and life, I have given and am still giving various lectures/workshops, in different countries and cultures. As I mentioned in the first part of this introduction, I am convinced that we are presently living at a most crucial historical juncture where the very best and the very worst is becoming more and more apparent and accessible to an ever-greater number of people. We are truly passing from "childhood" to "adulthood" by going through our collective "crisis of adolescence" when our culture and civilization are "touching bottom"; when we must pass from the horizontal to the vertical dimension; activate our intuition and awaken our spiritual consciousness so as to get in touch with our deeper self and with reality beyond the realm of mere appearances and phenomena.

This is not an easy period and life is becoming evermore demanding and stressful. To pass through this period (which we have chosen to live on earth as we were born at this particular time) we need not to *be judged* for our mistakes and follies but to *be helped* to take our next step forward and to pass through this transformation. Hence, most people living at this particular time will need all the resources and potentials, both internal and external, all the help they can get to make sense of their lives, discover who they really are and what they have come into this world to do. The realization that we are a *homo triplex*, a great spiritual being, who has incarnated in this material world to actualize his/her faculties and potentialities so as to accomplish the *Magnum Opus*, the Great Work; that we are an immortal rather than mortal beings; that we are not alone in this universe which is neither indifferent nor ruled by chance; and that we can get real help from the higher powers, both internal and external, but only once we have done and given all that we can . . . is *truly fundamental*!

Here religion and spirituality can each make truly essential and unique contributions upon which we must all draw, but in different ways, in order to live a truly conscious life which is what Life and Evolution now demand of all of us. And this implies to learn how to become responsible, autonomous, and productive, to live in a healthy and moral way, and be creative and joyful! But in order to accomplish this, to become an "endless mine" of insight, guidance, life, healing, and inspiration, the exoteric and esoteric aspects, the "letter" and the "spirit" of religion must be reunited and vivified; religion, the means, must be reunited with the end, spirituality. And this is what this book is all about. Bear in mind, however, that YOU, each of you, must do the *personal work required*, and that this book is but a set of guidelines, points of reference, and model for you to apply this perspective and use these instruments in you own personal and unique way.

The core insights, principles, ideas, and exercises contained in these materials should provide the perspective or theory (knowledge) and the practical exercises or experiments (the application and incarnation of this knowledge) to lead the serious and mature reader to draw the very best from one of the oldest and most important human institution: religion, which is the means, with its essential goal or end which is spirituality. Readers who will not only understand what these are and what they can do for them, but who will integrate them in their consciousness and being to live and incarnate them will then reap their highest fruit: provide a living example and find a model of what a human being can become and be at his/her very best. For we are not yet finished and completed beings, we are beings undergoing an evolution where, to a large extend, we can determine and become what we want and where we are, literally, *co-creators with God*, the Ultimate Reality!

As we move into the future, expand our human consciousness, actualize and utilize our faculties and potentialities, and thus create a new culture and civilization, we also multiply the problems and demands, the *stressors*, we are called to face and respond to. This means that the challenges to the human spirit, our survival instinct and our ability to perceive meaning and purpose in what are living are also increasing, both quantitatively and qualitatively! More than ever before, we need to be helped, not judged or condemned for all the mistakes and the crazy things we have done and are still doing; we need to face the truly essential questions of life, which are grossly neglected by our culture and universities, and be able to consciously tap our inner resources to understand what is happening and to cope with our problems.

We need to be able to answer the "riddle of the Sphinx": Who am I really (what is my true identity)? Where do I come from (what are my origins)? Where am I going (what is my destiny)? And what have I come to do in this world (what is my true vocation)? What are good and evil for me? How can I "discover" and consciously connect with the inexhaustible Source of Life, Love and Wisdom that already dwells within the depths of my being and in the heights of my consciousness? We need to understand what our relationship is to ourselves, to others, to Nature and to God. But we need to do this in a manner that is compatible with our present level of consciousness and being—with our present level of evolution.

Most important, we need a trans-empirical frame of reference that can lead us to the heart of reality (both internal and external) which our five senses and reason cannot possibly grasp and comprehend; we need to move beyond the finite and temporal physical world in which we now live to reach that which is infinite and eternal—which truly IS! And this has always been the province of religion! But religion, when it is authentic, needs to be properly understood and lived, which is not an easy thing and which requires much work, patience, perseverance and humility . . . for religion utilizes a special language and vocabulary that is dynamic, evolving and changing, as it is a function of our level of consciousness and being. It works with symbols, archetypes, myths, parables, and metaphors which appeal to our whole psyche and not just to the mind as does the language of science with its concepts and rational analyses.

This is why it is so important to have a proper understanding of religion: its nature, basic characteristics, inner dynamics and manifestations, and of its possible contributions and relationship to spirituality. In order to articulate a basic perspective or theory of religion, we are going to look at the seven major world religions, what they have in common, how they differ, and what might be their common core. Then we are going to look at the relationship of religion to spirituality to put both in proper focus and perspective. Finally, we are also going to see how religion and spirituality can be of theoretical and practical help to the modern man and woman in general and to the medical profession, to doctors and their patients in particular.

PART I

The Major World Religions

Introduction

THE BEGINNING OF THE JOURNEY

When I was very young I traveled a lot, as my family went to many places, in Europe first then also to Africa and South America. Somehow, I managed to structure my adult life in such a way that I could keep on traveling, something that I still do today when I should really be thinking about retirement! I can remember that the very first thing that really struck my conscious awareness as a child and that, in fact, hit me as the proverbial "ton of bricks" was just how much **suffering** there was in the world, not matter where we went or whom I spoke to! Life on earth for the vast majority of people everywhere seemed to be an "infinite ocean of diverse but very real suffering"! Thus, I asked myself two very basic questions:

- First, why is there so much suffering? What can be the cause, the nature, and the dynamics of human suffering?
- Second, can anyone, can I, do **anything** to alleviate that suffering?

My first reaction, as we visited and sojourned in very poor countries with many people living **below** the threshold of absolute (not relative) poverty, was *economic development*, the answer provided by the main axis of the United Nations, the UNDP. If, somehow, people could get trained, motivated, and guided to obtain better jobs or even a steady and dignified job, maybe a great deal of suffering would then disappear, so I thought in my youthful mind! We did, however, also have some very rich friends whom I knew quite well and it did not take me long to realize that they too have had many problems and pains, sufferings, but of a different kind. Hence, I concluded, while economic development is very important, it cannot answer the truly "essential" aspect of human suffering!

My next investigation took me to the world of *politics*. We had visited some countries that were real dictatorships, where those who had power and wealth could pretty much do as they pleased, putting themselves above the law with the literal power of "life and death" over many of their own people. Thus I thought that if only we could get a good constitution and rulers with integrity, justice, and compassion, then a great deal of suffering could, indeed, be avoided. So, I began to study political history but soon realized that, again, political reforms are very important but do not answer the root-cause of human suffering . . . as people continued to suffer in countries that had good governments and constitutions just as they did in those that had bad governments and constitutions, but in a different way.

So, I tried to continue my search and dug even deeper. To really understand and then attempt to answer the universal problem of human suffering, one must achieve self-knowledge, self-mastery, personal responsibility and a proper understanding of human nature, origins and destiny. This led me to *education, science and research*. Here at last, I thought, given enough time, good will, efforts, proper striving and the necessary means, we should be able to find the appropriate solutions! And so, I vowed to dedicate my life to education, science, and research, to obtain the knowledge and understanding, as well as the practical "skills and instruments" to answer that truly fundamental question. Time went by and more than 40 years later I am still dedicating most of my time, resources and energies, to education and research. More than two decades ago, however, I once more came to the conclusion that, important as this area and endeavor of human life is, it cannot provide the truly "soul-satisfying answer" I (and many other people as well) was looking for!

If economics, politics, science, education and research, cannot provide the answers to the most important questions human beings ask and to the problem of human suffering in particular, what can? Is it possible to find a truly satisfying answer that will bring with it the serenity, peace of mind and harmony that are so important and which, in different ways, we are all looking for? For quite a while, I did not think so, and I decided to slowly and humbly move in that direction through my own efforts, experiments, and research. One day, however, I had a very interesting conversation with a person who argued that Buddhism was designed to specifically answer that question and addressed itself to the understanding and elimination of human suffering.

That, immediately, brought my attention to **religion** and the possibility that it might have the answers I was looking for. After further investigation, experimentation, and reflection I finally concluded that religion does, indeed, have these answers; however, not the popular "exoteric" form of religion but, rather, its "esoteric" version, the religion of the Saints and Sages, of those who have *awakened their spiritual consciousness*! Hence, my life-long work and interest in "esoteric" or "mystical" religion; in spirituality and spiritual consciousness and their possibilities and potentialities in particular; and in the religion of the Saints and Sages (or, better put, in their interpretation and application of a given religion) to answer many fundamental questions and problems—that of holistic health, peace, and serenity, as well as happiness, in particular.

Chapter I

WHAT HUMAN BEINGS REALLY
WANT, THE ANSWER OF RELIGION

After a great deal of reflection and research, I concluded, as many other thinkers had before me, that science can make great contributions to minor questions while religion can make minor contributions to great questions! Rather than focusing upon and limiting myself to understand the nature, dynamics, and *raison d'être* of human suffering, I now plunged into the study of, and experimentation with, even more fundamental questions that would provide the proper perspective to understand human suffering: what it really is and what we can do about it. These are:

- What is a human being: his nature, origins, destiny, and duty in this world?
- What is the universe, who or what created the universe, and for what purpose?
- What is Life, who or what created Life and for what purpose?
- Can a human being truly solve the enigma of human life and of the human condition and thus achieve true and lasting peace, health, joy, and fulfillment while incarnate in this world?

In the present and the chapters that will follow, I will seek to answer these questions and to share with you my most basic assumptions, conclusions as well as the theoretical perspective and practical instruments of the spiritual tradition for doing so.

Recently, I came across a book by a truly inspired person and great American philosopher, Huston Smith, who for many years taught Philosophy at M.I.T., entitled *The Religions of Man*. Besides its clarity, insight, and succinctness, this work focused in particular upon how the most important religions (Hinduism, Buddhism, Confucianism, Taoism, Islam, Judaism, and Christianity) defined the essential *needs* and *aspirations* of man and how they sought to answer them. This was the main "springboard" and frame of reference for the first part of this book, "what human beings really want" and how do different religions, spiritual and philosophical systems perceive and define the critical human *needs* and *aspirations,* and how do they go about satisfying them. These answers can be applied to the "exoteric" as well as to the "esoteric" aspects and on the various levels of consciousness and being with varying interpretations, implications, applications and nuances.

The beauty and usefulness of this approach, at least for me, is that it fully recognized what I termed and researched as the "human sky-scraper" theory and the analogy of the "vertical axis of consciousness": the fact that what we call "Reality" and "Truth" are really *functions of our level of consciousness and being.* This I consider truly fundamental in that it explains why people do not perceive, define, want, or pursue the same values and goals and which make up the inescapable differences, contradictions, and paradoxes of human life. It also points to the fact that human beings have an **organic** growth and development which means that they must **live** and cannot **skip** any of the basic stages or phases of human becoming or evolution. Let us then begin our journey and exploration by looking at *Hinduism,* one of the oldest religions of humankind; what it can tell us and what we can learn from it; for it can prepare us for our religious, spiritual, and philosophical adventure in a very simple and practical way that takes us to what is really essential and practical and, therefore, *useful.*

Chapter II

HINDUISM

Hinduism is a compendium of various realizations (in higher levels of consciousness) and traditions, experienced by Saints and Sages over a long period of time which coalesced to form one of the oldest and most spiritual religions of humanity. Looking at what is known as "Hinduism" as a whole, its vast and complex literature, exotic art, complex rituals, and elaborate folklore and condensing it into one, very simple but extremely profound, affirmation, we would find that it is saying to all human beings: *in time you can have what you want!* Other traditions and approaches have said and repeated the same thing, but in different words. Probably, the best version is "be careful what you truly pray for and desire because that is what you will, eventually, *get* and then *have to live with!*" But what do people truly want?

1. **They want pleasure**. This is very natural and instinctive as we are all born and endowed with pleasure/pain sensibilities. This is our first and most basic motivational system that very clearly and loudly tell us what is "good" (pleasure) and was "bad" (pain) so that we will seek the first and try to avoid the second. Moreover, the world is filled with incredibly diversified possibilities for enjoyment. The sensory world is replete with beauty and delights for our senses and there are other levels and dimensions (the emotional, mental, and spiritual) that hold even greater and far more intense gratification. Hedonism, like everything else, calls for *balance* and *harmony*: too much or too little, too soon or too late, would spoil the effect so it is prudent to sacrifice small, immediate rewards for greater future ones. Far from condemning pleasure, Hinduism points to how we have increase it and experience it to the fullest possible extent, provided that we do not become *addicted* to any of its forms and do not *harm* others or ourselves (violate moral

principles). Does this sound familiar? St. Paul already had declared, a long time ago that "you can have and do what you want, but everything has its consequences". Today, its basic expression is: "Do whatever will make you happy provided it does not harm others" and which is what many people, in fact do, whether they are conscious of it or not!

2. Then, comes **worldly success** in its three basic aspects of **wealth, fame** and **power**. Here, we have the Gospel not of *sensualism* but of *success* which has conquered the West and the Anglo-American world in particular. These run deep and should not be disparaged for they enable us to survive and discharge our civic duties, to bring a sense of dignity and self respect, to create cosmos out of chaos in the world and in ourselves, and seem to feed our ego as nothing else can and thus to "launch us" on the great journey and adventure of Life on earth.

Taken together, the above constitute what Hinduism called "the way of Desire", the "wisdom of men" or the fulfillment of the needs and aspirations of the human ego which are always short-term, sensual, egoistical, and hedonistic in nature. In contrast and opposition to the "Path of Desire" is the "Way of Renunciation", the "wisdom of God", or the fulfillment of the needs and aspirations of the human soul and Self which are always long-term, spiritual, holistic, and truly fulfilling. The Hindu word for the full self-actualization and Self-realization of Man, for the return to his Source and Essence, is *yoga* which comes from the same etymological root as the word "yoke" that has two basic connotations: *to unite* or bring together and to *place under a discipline* or training; it is the equivalent of the Greek word *askesis* which gave us the word ascetic and asceticism. There are, naturally, many "yogas" but four are the truly essential ones: *karma yoga*, the way of work, *jnana yoga*, the way of knowledge, *bhaki yoga*, the way of love, and *raja yoga*, the way of spiritual exercises.

Hinduism has always believed in both the *immortality of the soul* and in multiple lives on earth—in *reincarnation*. Hence, it comes very close to and implicitly recognizes my image of the "human sky-scraper" and of the "vertical axis of consciousness"; namely that not all people function on the same level of consciousness, being, and evolution, and that there are different "types of people", or people with different evolutionary ages, who walk and live in the physical world. Most people in the world are still "babies", "infants", and "adolescents", even though there have always been a few "adults" in our midst as well. Today, what we are witnessing in the world and in our environment is what I call the passage from "the man of talent", the adolescent, to the "disciple", the young adult, which entails a new and higher level of consciousness and way of perceiving, defining, and reacting to the same things.

In terms of the above perspective, the "Path of Desire", pleasure and worldly success, is the way of children and adolescents who like to play games, experiment with everything and to invent ever new and more diverse toys. There is nothing intrinsically wrong with that and it may well be that everyone must "pass through and live this stage". It is equally clear, however, that the "Path of Desire", the "wisdom of men", and the gratification of the ego, is *inadequate* and *temporary*. The world's visible and sensual pleasures and gratifications never truly satisfy a person so that that person will always want more of them and thus there will come a time (which for me is our historical juncture) when that person will be caught on a tread mill, having to race faster and faster for rewards that mean less and less! These rewards are also ephemeral and will never "endure forever", which is what people, who are truly happy, really want! Finally, they are also *exclusive*, hence competitive, scarce, and conflictual. Hence, pleasure, wealth, power, and fame are really the "toys" of children which will someday be outgrown.

The "Path of Renunciation", the "wisdom of God", or the way of the soul and of the Self, always involves growth and self-transcendence, hence discipline, efforts, training, self-knowledge and self-mastery as any art would require. Here an analogy may be helpful: if you want to climb to the top of a mountain (regeneration) being one quarter of the way there, you must know what you want, discipline yourself, and make efforts to continue climbing. Whereas, if you want to go back down to the foot of the mountain (degeneration), all you have to do is to let yourself go, follow the path of least resistance, and "slide down the slope"! For Hinduism, what people really want is *union with their true Self and with Reality,* the fullest actualization of all their potentialities and faculties, and there are four basic paths that lead there, depending on your type of consciousness and level of evolution. These are:

3. **The way of work, duty and integrity,** which they call *karma yoga.* As a well-known physician once remarked, "the human machine seems to be made for work". Work is the staple of life and, without it, no one could survive or grow. Hence, you do not have to retire to a cloister to find God; you can find Him in the world as readily as anywhere! The key here is to throw yourself into your work with everything you have but do so *wisely* and in a way that will bring out the highest rewards consonant with your destiny. The real secret of work is to do it *for God* rather than for *oneself* or for the social and economic rewards it can bring. Thus, whatever you do, do as well as you can: do your best in every thing you undertake, or don't do it; do *your best*, not less and not more as harmony is truly essential". This in turn, will develop your will and lead you to the "heroic path" as it is known in the Western tradition, the way of self-expression and creation. The essential goal and objective here being to go beyond and transcend the smallness of the finite human self and discover and unite with the true, infinite, spiritual Self.

4. **The way of knowledge or understanding**, which they call *jnana yoga*. For Hinduism, this is the path to oneness with the Godhead through mental and intellectual effort. It appeals particularly to people who are intellectuals and who has a philosophical bent. Socrates and the Buddha are good examples of those who have used this path. The central aim of this approach is to "cleave the domain of ignorance with the sword of discernment and inspiration". What is required here is to be able to see beyond the surface and the shadow of reality, and thus of the human ego, to what is truly *real* and thus *meaningful*. In the Western tradition is path is known as the "Gnostic path" or the "occult path".

5. **The way of love or mysticism**, which they call *bhakti yoga*. For most people, life is fueled not so much by reason as by emotions. The most powerful and pervasive of these is "love". Even hatred can be looked at as the "dark side of love" when love has been thwarted or betrayed. Moreover, men tend to become like that which they love. Thus, the aim of bhakti yogi is to direct towards God the geyser of love that lies at the root of the human heart. As the *Bhagavata Purana* succinctly puts it: "As the waters of the Ganges flow incessantly toward the ocean, so do the minds of the bhaktas move constantly toward Me, the supreme Person residing in every heart, immediately they hear about My qualities." This is the most popular and, in my opinion, the deepest and most authentic of the four paths and the one generally associated with Christianity.

As Huston Smith incisively put it: "In *jnana yoga* the guiding image was an infinite sea of being underlying the tiny waves of our finite selves. God was thought as an all-pervading Self, as fully present within us as without. The task was to recognize our identity with Him. Moreover, God was conceived primarily in impersonal terms, for the characteristic of ultimate reality that most impresses the philosopher is His infinity in comparison with which personality, embodying as it must certain properties to the exclusion of others, must always seem in some respects a limitation. For one to whom love means more than mind, God must appear different on each of these counts. First, as love when healthy is an out-turning emotion, the bhakti will reject all suggestion that the God he loves is himself, even the deepest Self, and insist on His Otherness . . . "I want to taste sugar; I don't want to be sugar!"

Then, he concludes, "His aim will not be to perceive his identity with God but to adore Him with every element of his being . . . This union . . . is no pantheistic absorption of the man in the one . . . but is essentially *personal* in character . . . More, since it is preeminently a *union of love*, the kind of knowledge which is required is that of *friendship* in the very highest sense of the word . . . . In such a context, God's personality far from being a limitation is indispensable. Philosophers may be able to love pure being, infinite beyond all attributes, but they are exceptions. The normal object of human love is *personality*, however exalted its attributes of wisdom, compassion, and grace may be."

6. **The way of psychospiritual exercises** or *raja yoga*. Because of the heights to which it can lead and the speed at which it does so, this path is known as "the royal road to reintegration or Self-realization". Designed for persons who are basically "scientific or "logico-empirical" in bent, it is the way to God through psychological experiment. The West has often honored the empiricist in the laboratory but distrusted him in the affairs of the spirit! India has no such fears; the affairs of the spirit can be experimented with just as well as those of nature. As Huston Smith concludes, "All that is required is a strong suspicion that our true selves are vastly more wonderful than we realize, and a passion for *direct experience* of their full reach . . . . Given a basically spiritual orientation and outreach, however, all that is proposed is that the yogi undertakes a series of experiments with all the patience and rigor of a frontier experiment in physics and carefully observes the outcome."

Unlike the experiments of Western science that deal with the outer, physical world, the experiments of raja yoga deal with human nature, human consciousness and the spirit. Essentially, these experiments take the form of utilizing certain psychospiritual exercises and then observing the effects of these on one's consciousness and being.

Finally, Hinduism also conceives of "four basic stages of life" during which the needs, aspirations, and duties of a human being change radically. First, we have the stage of the **child** and **student** wherein one learns about one's self, the world, and one's calling in the world. Here one has to acquire both the knowledge and skills to live, or survive, and to accomplish one's destiny or "duty" (*dharma*). The second stage, which begins with marriage, is that of the **householder**: the creation of a family, work in the world, and turning one's attention and energies outwardly. This is followed by the stage of **retirement** which generally comes with the arrival of the first grandchild. This is the time when the individual frees himself from the requirements society and begins his true adult education—to discover who he really is and what life is all about. What is the real secret of his identity and destiny? The business of education, family, occupation, secular life is left behind and only eternity remains! The fourth and final stage, in which the ultimate goal is actually achieved or not, is that of the **sannyasin**. The Bhagavad-Gita defines it as "one who neither hates nor love anything". One is free to return to the world but not for the sake of the world or as the "homeless mendicant" but as one who is completely free to truly *be himself!*

What do human beings really want? They want to avoid pain and seek pleasure (Freud), they want the power to be and to express themselves (Adler), they want to find meaning and purpose in their lives (Jung and Frankel). They want different things at different stages of their evolution and becoming, at different points of their life-cycles, and in different cultures and socio-historical conditions. Most of them don't know what they really want: they are searching, groping, and exchanging one thing or passion for another.

Abraham Maslow developed and proposed his well-known "hierarchy of needs": first, human beings want to survive biologically by being able to satisfy their physical needs (thus money); then, they seek security at the physical and emotional level (hence, the ability to continue to meet their physical needs in time); then, they seek affection, the ability to give, receive, and experience *love*; then, they want the esteem and recognition of others (social status); finally, they want self-actualization (the full development and expression of their latent faculties and potentialities).

Greek mythology suggested that what human beings, after having experienced and experimented with various gratifications of their ego, really want is to discover "who they really are", that is, "answer the riddle of the Sphinx" (Who am I? Where do I come from? Where am I going, and what have I come to do in this world?) or what modern psychology calls the problem of identity, origins, destiny, and calling.

Hinduism, which is one of the oldest, most profound and comprehensive, religions argued exactly what I have concluded, namely that "what human beings really want" is a function of their level of consciousness and being and thus will vary with their level of evolution, their biological age, and their sociocultural conditions and personal experiences. Clearly, they want pleasure (and thus to avoid pain), they want security, wealth, power, and fame, love and knowledge especially self-knowledge! But, in the end, they want union with themselves and with reality, the fullest possible actualization of their potentialities and the realization of their true Self, which is traditionally known as "union with God". With a foundation in psychological and moral balance, Hinduism suggested that people can achieve what they want (when they finally discover what it truly is!) through work, personal character and integrity, knowledge, love, and psychospiritual exercises.

What do **you want** at the present stage of your life? And how do you feel you can answer and achieve what you truly want? This is the final and most important question and a question to which *you* are the only one that can really answer it! Whatever you will find in the world, other people, models and examples, traditions and religions, are merely a "mirror" and a set of "guide-lines" to help you answer this fundamental question which is preeminently a *personal question* and one which each individual must find the answer to through his/her own personal experience! Let us not forget the wonderful saying of the mystic Angelus Silesius, "If Jesus were to be born a thousand times in Bethlehem but not in your own soul, you would not be saved!"

Chapter III

CONFUCIANISM

If there is one name with which Chinese culture has been associated and which helped to fashion and forge it, it is that of Confucius—Kung Fu-Tzu or Kung, the Master. The Chinese (with the exception of the Communists!) reverently speak of him as the "First Teacher"! No one claims that he molded Chinese culture all by himself, he least of all as he was wont to depreciate his innovations and regard himself as a "lover of the ancients". Another very important person who left a deep imprint upon Chinese culture, brought about a new religion, and complemented Confucianism is Lao Tzu, the "Old Boy", or "Grand Master" (the meaning of his name in Chinese) who was responsible for articulating what became known as Taoism.

We shall look first at the person, life, and teaching of the first and then of the second. Basically, Confucianism and Taoism blended and integrated the *yin and yang*: the masculine and feminine, the active and passive, the inner and the outer, the classical and romantic, and the "this-worldly" and "other-worldly" aspect of Chinese culture, tradition and religion. Hence, they must be seen within the same overall perspective and philosophical framework with the understanding that polarity and opposites can and must be reconciled.

Confucius was born around 551 B.C. in the Province now known as Shantung. Little is known about his family except that it was not wealthy or with social standing and that his father died when he was three years old. The financial hardship of his youth gave him a feeling for the common people which was reflected in the democratic and compassionate traits of his philosophy. At the age of 15, he focused upon *education* and *learning* which became the supreme values of his life. After holding several small government posts and contracting a not too successful marriage, he established himself as a *tutor* (first of individuals and than of states) which became his vocation.

His main concern and thrust was "this-worldly", thus *social action* and *politics*. His goal was *public office* in that he firmly believed that his insights and theories would not be understood and useful unless applied to the world of human affairs through public administration. He had a supreme faith in his ability to reorder society and bring about peace, justice, and happiness to the many. Being told about the strong growth of population in his state of Wei and asked what could be done about this he answered, "Enrich them by educating them". Later in his life, for a brief period of time, he did achieve high political positions including Minister of Public Works, of Justice, and even Prime Minister! The primary virtues he advocated in men were *loyalty* and *good will* while in women it was *chastity* and *docility*.

All genuine religions have always had two central axes at the very core of their theory and practice: the *love of God* (prayer, worship, and contemplation) and the *love of our fellow humans* (social action, political and economic development). The first culminated in mysticism and Self-realization while the second in justice and self-actualization. Confucianism privileged the first while Taoism the second. The key to social justice and peace is always *personal virtue* thus, for Confucius, we should always learn how to govern ourselves before we seek to govern others. This was his most important advice, together with honesty and truthfulness, for the individual and the ruler alike. It was only when he reached his 50's that he became fully aware of his "divine mission" and that he pursued it by wandering from state to state in the "long trek" to improve both life on earth and the actualization of human potentials. Only self-discipline, strenuous effort, and proper organization would offset the "ills of a society beyond redemption"! Chinese peasants saw him the "the man who knows he cannot succeed but keeps on trying"!

Confucius died at the age of 73 about 479 B.C. teaching and publishing the classics. While a failure as a politician, he was undoubtedly one of the world's greatest teachers who managed to meet the other most influential person in China, a teacher in his own lifetime, Lao Tzu. Like Socrates, he was a one-man university, always informal and seeking to bring out answers to the fundamental questions of earthly life from the depths of the other persons' consciousness. He remained always more exacting of himself that of others and was quite *this-worldly* in his approach which consisted in doing, experiencing, and enjoying everything *in moderation*. Power and wealth could have been his had he been willing to compromise with those in authority, but he always preferred his own integrity and good conscience. Confucius developed a series of aphorisms, known as *The Analects*, which contain the essence of his thought. Some of the best known ones are:

"What you do not wish done to yourself, do not do to others"; "Do not wish for quick results, nor look for small advantages. If you seek quick results, you will not attain the ultimate goal. If you are led astray by small advantages, you will never accomplish great things"; "If, when you look into your own heart, you find nothing wrong there, what is there to worry about, what is there to fear?"; "A man without virtue cannot long abide in adversity, nor can he abide long in happiness"; "Wealth and rank are what men desire, but unless they be obtained in the right way they cannot be possessed".

To understand Confucius' power and influence, we must put both his life and teachings in the perspective of the place and time in which he lived. In a nutshell, this was the problem of social anarchy! In those days, there were no Kings in China and every person did what they wanted and felt was right in their own eyes. What holds living creatures together, the pack, the herd, is *instinct*. With the birth of Man, this natural source of cohesion weakens and disappears, for Man is the "animal without instincts". So what is to keep anarchy and anomie in check? What has been called the "cake of custom", values and behavioral patterns that have emerged and worked over a long period of time. With the passage of time and evolution, reason replaced social habit and self-interest prevailed over the expectations of the group. "What's in it for me" became the key question! Individualism and self-consciousness are contagious: once they emerge they continue to spread and the unreflecting oneness of the group is gone.

When tradition is no longer adequate to hold society together, man faces a very serious crisis. America is one of the most tradition-less societies we know of. As a substitute it proposed *reason*. Educate people and provide them with the facts can use to make rational decisions and people will behave sensibly and well. This has been the Jeffersonian-Enlightenment creed on which America proceeded. But it has paid a price for this—rising crime, divorce, psychopathology, depression, and delinquency rates! Two basic approaches developed to cope with this truly fundamental problem: that of the Realists and that of the Idealists. For the Realists, the problem of social order can be solved with "laws with teeth in them". Ultimately what people understand and which works best is *physical force*.

The Idealists, whose main proponent was Mo Tzu, argued that the real solution of the social problem was not force but *love*. The only real hope for peace lay in brotherly kindness and good will toward all. Underpinning both positions stood an opposed view of the universe. The Realists thought that it was either indifferent or hostile to human beings whereas the Idealists postulated that the Creator of the universe, *Shang Ti*, was essentially good. As love is obviously good and the God who created and governs the world is good, it is inconceivable that He would have made a world in which love did not pay off! Confucius saw positive and negatives in both positions which he considered to be only half a solution! Confucius also thought that reason, however developed and refined, would, in the end, prove to be only an instrument for rationalized *self-interest*. Confucius was a student and a lover of the past. He saw a Grand

Harmony to have ruled the world and society (China) until men had become individuals, self-conscious and self-seeking.

To really work, a solution to the social problem must meet two basic conditions: preserve true continuity and answer the most pressing present problems. Confucius appealed to the classics which he reinterpreted for his contemporary generation, thus shifting tradition from an unconscious to a conscious orientation. To shift from spontaneous to deliberate tradition, required the powers of *critical intelligence*, which he sought to unfold in himself and in his followers, to preserve tradition and to define its present objectives. So Confucius' task was to create the prototype of what Chinese national character could be—that of a sage or of a "gentleman". Deliberate tradition differs from spontaneous tradition in that it requires *attention, focus* and *effort*.

The essential Confucian doctrine rested upon five master concepts and their interrelations which are:

1. *Jen*, etymologically speaking this is a combination of the characters for "man" and for "good relationship". Thus, it implies "good will", "benevolence", and "the dignity and value of human life". As it brings together self-respect and compassion and care for others, it is the virtue of virtues and the mainspring for all the other concepts. For Confucius it is in *Jen* that can be found the perfection of everything that separates human beings from animals; thus he stated, "in public life the man of *Jen* is untiringly diligent and in his private life, courteous, unselfish, and gifted with empathy. Its ultimate significance is that all human beings are brothers and related to each other".

2. *Chun-tzu*. While *Jen* points to the "right relationship" between people, *Chun-tzu* shows the goal of the former: the fully developed or "superior man", man-at-its-best. It is the equivalent of the English "gentleman" and of the French "chevalier", the opposite of the petty, uncouth, self-centered person. It is the person who is now at home in the universe and who can truly say "nothing that is human will be alien to me".

3. *Li,* which means propriety, *savoir faire*, manners. It was his conception and blue-print for the making of the Chinese national character. It deals directly with basic postulates of the Rectification of Names (words should always relate to something in reality and not exist for themselves or distort reality); the Mean (harmony or proper proportions); the Five Relationships (these make up the warp of Chinese social life and include the relationship between father and son, elder brother and younger brother, husband and wife, older friend and younger friend, and ruler and subject); the Family (in this approach, the family is the basic unit of society and what brought the Chinese from the animal

to the human level; and finally Age (the great respect for age that has always characterized Chinese culture and manners).

4. *Te.* Literally, this means "power" and more specifically the power through which men are ruled. Power, however, here involves moral as well as physical power. Keep in mind Napoleon's famous saying "God is always on the side that has the strongest battalions" to which his Foreign Minister, Talleyrand, replied, "One can do everything with bayonets . . . except sit on them"! Real, enduring power always lies in *moral example* in that if people have no trust in their government and its leaders it cannot last long! Like Thomas Jefferson, Confucius would have argued, "The whole art of government consists in the art of being honest".

5. *Wen* which implies the "arts of peace" as opposed to the "arts of war": literature, philosophy, poetry, and the arts. The ultimate victory, Confucius, argued, always goes to the state that develops the most exalted and complete *culture*—the finest arts, the noblest philosophy, and the greatest poetry!

Thus, goodness, the gentleman, good manners, virtuous government, and the flourishing of the arts constitute the heart and core of the Confucian doctrine. In his own words and in an aphorismic expression: "If there be righteousness in the heart, there will be beauty in the character. If there is beauty in the character, there will be harmony in the home. If there is harmony in the home, there will be order in the nation. If there is order in the nation, then there will be peace in the world". This is the teachings that Confucius brought together and promulgated as education: a philosophy and art of living. It brought "down to earth" the earlier religious tradition of China which was quite animistic, ancestor-oriented, and abstract.

Here, Heaven and earth were seen as being on a continuum with human beings right in the middle, the "Middle Kingdom". Heaven was composed of the ancestors and was ruled by *Shang Ti*, the supreme ancestor. The ancestors would soon be joined by those now alive on earth so that death was really a "promotion" to a more honorable estate by those who had lived honorably and with integrity. Thus Heaven was more important than Earth as their inhabitants were more venerable and their authority greater. Hence they commanded those living on earth and dominated their imagination. Sacrifice was the way in which Earth related to Heaven and augury was the language that united the two as ancestor's worship was the way to remain connected. Confucius, however, shifted the emphasis from Heaven to Earth but without dropping Heaven out of the picture altogether, seeking to distill the best from both but putting the accent on the "here and now"!

Basically, his philosophy was an incarnation and objectification of *common sense* and *pragmatic wisdom*. Whenever he was questioned about the other world, Confucius always brought back the focus to this world. When asked about the spirit of the dead, he replied, "While you are not able to serve men, how can you serve their spirits?" And when asked about death, he states, "While you do not know life, how can you know anything about death?" Finally, he also changed the emphasis from ancestor worship to filial piety—hence to Earth rather than Heaven. However, he also stated one of the most often quoted religious aphorisms, "He who offends the gods has no one to whom he can pray!"

To sum up the Confucian doctrine in one sentence, it would be "The ideal of life on earth is a social order in communion cooperation with a cosmic order: Man and Nature are inseparable". In China it was age that was accorded the greatest attention and veneration in opposition to the youth-orientation of America. In social prestige, it is the scholar that traditionally ranked at the top of the scale and the soldier at the bottom. Acute social sensitivity, which Confucius used to transmit tradition, was manifested in the concept of "saving face" or one's honor and that of one's family. Genuine prophets have a strange way of outlasting politicians and educators. Thus as Jesus outlasted Herod, Gandhi Nehru, so will Confucius outlast Mao Tze-Tung! Confucius was a true Prophet and authentic Sage who reflected the level of consciousness and the culture of his time.

Chapter IV

TAOISM

Lao Tzu was born around 604 B.C., about half a century before Confucius. Legends have sprung around his birth arguing that he was immaculately conceived, that his mother carried him in her womb for more than 80 years, and that he was born already wise, an old man with a beard! Disappointed with the impact of his teachings, it was said that Lao Tzu climbed on a water buffalo and moved to Tibet. His literary testament and the heart of his doctrine can be found in a very small book entitled *"Tao Te Ching"* or the way of nature and its power. It is a hymn to man's place and home in the universe and can be read and reflected upon in half an hour . . . or in a life-time!

Tao is the master concept which, literally, means the "path" or the "way". It has, however, three essential levels of meanings:

1. *It is the way of ultimate reality* and, as such, cannot be perceived by the senses. Should it reveal itself in its full glory and power, it would blind us. It also cannot be grasped by the emotions, thoughts, or imagination. Whence we have the two well-known aphorisms: "The Tao that can be conceived is not the real Tao" and "Those who know do not speak and those who speak do not know". But, while the Tao is transcendent, it is also immanent.

2. *It is the way of the universe*: the principle, the energy, and the rhythm in all nature, the ordering principle behind all life. When the Tao incarnates and "assumes material expression", it adapts and regulates all things. As such it can be seen as the "Mother of the World" and likened to Bergson's *élan vital* as well as to the *lex aeterna* of classical philosophy.

3. *It is the way in which man should order his life* . . . so as to be in harmony with the universe and with himself.

In Ancient China, three very different types of Taoism have developed: the magical, the mystical, and the philosophical. According to these three ways, *Te*, or power, can be approached as "magical", which formed the core of popular Taoism. Here spirituality becomes mystification and religion is perverted into necromancy and sorcery. Or it can be approached as "mystical" which gave rise to "esoteric Taoism". The power that holds society together is neither "magical" (popular Taoism) nor moral example (Confucianism) but essentially *psychospiritual* in nature. Thus a few exceptional individuals (Saints and Sages) in each community could become the living receptacles for the Tao and radiate a healing, inspiring, and vivifying energy over the place they lived and the people that came in contact with them. In opposition to Confucianism, Taoism was fascinated by and privileged the *inner* rather than the *outer* man.

Successive deposits of toil, passion, and worry had so darkened the soul (the "Fall") that it was necessary to work backwards through these layers until "the original man, man-as-he-was-supposed-to-be" could emerge. Pure consciousness would then be accessed that would reveal Spirit. To arrive at this higher level of consciousness, it was necessary to end self-seeking, egoism, and greed, and to cultivate perfect cleanliness of thought, emotion, and body. Pure Spirit can only reveal itself when all is purified and cleansed. Thus, selflessness, cleanliness, and emotional serenity are the essential preliminaries to reach full self-knowledge that can only be revealed by the Spirit, and then will follow truth, power, and joy and everything that man has ever sought! The central aphorism of Taoism is thus, "To the mind that is still the whole universe surrenders".

Philosophical Taoism argues that there is a third way of looking at the Tao which is neither magical nor mystical but philosophical and psychological. Here, the way of the universe manifests itself to the mind that has purified itself and that is still. What is needed is neither spiritual nor psychic power but reflective, *rational power*. The essential quality of life manifested everywhere by the universe is *wu wei*, or "letting go", "creative quietness". This integrates in the person who has realized it two opposed conditions: supreme activity and supreme relaxation. *Wu wei* is the supreme action that occurs in "letting go and letting God", as we would put it. It is the freedom, simplicity, life and inspiration that flow from the core of our being and of the universe if we but let it manifest itself.

While Confucianism sought to generate a complete pattern of ideal conscious responses that might be imitated by others, Taoism sought the opposite: to allow the Tao that already is, both within us and within the universe, to *manifest itself*. Here action follows being rather than being emerging from action. Today and expressed in simpler words, this could be seen as *instruction* that comes from without, that must be learned and *education* that comes from within, that emerges from the depths of one's being! As the *Tao Te Ching* put it in a nutshell: "The way to do is simply . . . *to be*".

The best graphic representation of the Tao is *water*. The Chinese character for "swimmer" is "the one who knows the nature of water". So the Taoist adept is one who knows the nature of the basic *life-force* that will sustain him in all of life's vicissitudes. This is best represented in the following aphorism: "Those who flow as life flows know they need no other force. They feel no wear, they feel no tear, they need not mending nor repair." Water, then, is the best analogue of the Tao in the natural world and the prototype of *wu wei*. Another aphorism states: "Man is at his best, like water, serves as he goes along: like water he seeks his own level, the common level of Life". A final characteristic of water is the clarity it reaches through being clean and still. "Muddy water let stand . . . and it will clear", says the *Tao Te Ching*.

Following the image of water, Taoists reject all forms of self-assertiveness and competition as well as of strenuous effort and prolonged training. The world is full of people who are killing themselves and others to "be someone" or to attain success. They want to get ahead and stand out from the crowd. Taoism has little sympathy or respect for that attitude as it claims that "the ax always falls first on the tallest tree"! They also are strictly opposed to violence and verge on strict pacifism. This is why they claim that "In time of war men civilized in peace turn from their higher to their lower nature . . . He who thinks triumph beautiful is one with a will to kill. The death of a multitude is cause for mourning: conduct your triumph as a funeral." Their almost reverential attitude towards simplicity, naturalness, and humility led them to honor hunchbacks and cripples because of the way in which they represented meekness, self-effacement, and the acceptance of their lot. The Taoists refusal to strive for position and standing sprang from a profound disinterest in the things of this world. Thus for them, man should avoid being strident and aggressive towards other human beings and towards nature, who should be befriended and treated as relatives!

It was the drive towards simplicity and naturalness that most divided the Taoists from the Confucians. For the former, pomp and extravagances were regarded as pointless accretions for the later it was art and improvement. Another core value of Taoism is the notion of the relativity of all values and the integration of opposites. This can be clearly seen in core symbol of Taoism integrating the *yang yin* polarities. This polarity sums up all of life's paradoxes and oppositions: good-evil, active-passive, positive-negative, light-darkness, life-death, inner-outer, male-female, etc. These complement and counterbalance each other. Each enters into the other's field and goes to the center of the opposite's field. In the end both are resolved in an all-embracing circle, symbol of the final unity of life and of the Tao. Life does not move onward and forward toward a fixed pinnacle or goal; rather it "turns and bends back upon itself until the self comes full circle and knows that at the center, all things are *one*".

All values, concepts and ideas, insights and ideals are thus relative to the person who entertains them and to his level of consciousness and being.

Hence, no perspective in this world can be considered as *absolute*. No one knows when the longest way around to a given objective might not turn out to be the shortest way home. As Huston Smith put it: "That in traditional China the scholar ranked at the top of the social scale may be the doing of Confucius, but Taoism is fully responsible for placing the soldier at the bottom!" And he concluded, "Only the man who recognizes all men as members of his own body is a sound man to guard them . . . Heaven arms with compassion those whom she would not see destroyed".

Thus, "blending the *yang* and the *yin* in themselves", Taoism and Confucianism represent the two distinctive poles of Chinese religion and philosophy. "Confucius represents the classical, Lao Tzu the romantic. Confucius represents social responsibility; Lao Tzu sings the glories of spontaneity and naturalness. Confucius' focus is always on man, Lao Tzu beyond man . . . Confucius roams within society, Lao Tzu wanders beyond. Something in life reaches out in each of these directions, and Chinese civilization would certainly have been poorer if either had not emerged."

Chapter V

BUDDHISM

Buddhism, like many but not all religions, began with a man, with a very special man, who felt he had discovered *who he was* and what was the true answer to the human condition—to *human suffering*! Many times, as with Jesus of Nazareth, people asked him: "Who are you? Are you a God? Are you an Angel? Are you a Saint?" His answer was always, "no"! Finally, he told them, "I am awake" (i.e. I have become a *conscious being*!) and this is what Buddhism is really all about: *awakening*, raising one's level of consciousness and being to the point where one can begin to *live consciously*. In fact, in Sanskrit the root *buhd* means "to wake up, to know". So, the Buddha is the person who has awakened, the enlightened one, what we are all meant to become at the end of our earthly journey once we have reached human and spiritual maturity.

Interestingly enough, Jesus said the same thing but in different words, "I am the Son of Man", which is what *you* are meant to become when you reach your full human and spiritual maturity. Thus, in this sense, both Jesus and Buddha are an *archetype* and a *prototype* of what we are all destined to become, a "model" of the fully actualized, awakened, and realized human being who is truly *himself* and able to manifest the Spirit *consciously* in all of creation, of which the material world is but a small part, and of which they have become a "temple" or a "vehicle of expression".

For Buddhism the great majority of human beings are still unconscious, asleep, and immature—they are children who don't know *who* they are and *what* they came in the world to do. Thus, they are playing games, dangerous and painful games, (as with warfare, industrialization, commercial agriculture and allopathic healthcare, to mention only the better known ones). Buddhism began with an individual, with one Man, Siddhartha Gautama of the Sakyas (Siddhartha was his name, Gautama his surname, and Sakya the name of his clan), who shed the daze and doze of the dream-like existence of most human beings like the philosopher of the platonic cave who realized that most people look at the shadows on a cave rather than the sunlight! His destiny and mission was to show human beings what they really are and what they can become as they grow up.

Like that of Jesus, his life soon became a legend and myth: the blind received their sight, the deaf and dumb heard and started speaking, the crooked became straight, and the lame walked. Prisoners were freed from their chains and the fires of pain and despair of hell were quenched; even the brutality of the beasts ceased as peace and joy came to the earth . . . Historically, Gautama was born about 560 B.C. near Benares in Northern India. His father was the king of a small region or what we might call a "feudal Lord". He was very rich and beautiful and at the age of 16 he married a princess by the name of Yasodhara who gave him a son, Rahula. Thus, he was a man who had *everything* the world had to offer: noble birth, health, beauty, fame, power, money, intelligence, a lovely family and human love. In spite or perhaps *because* of this, in his early twenties he became restless and dissatisfied—he experienced "divine discontent". Thus he left his worldly station and radically changed his life.

At his birth, we are told, fortunetellers predicted that Gautama would either unify India and become its greatest King (achieve the pinnacle of temporal power) or, if he chose a spiritual path, that he would become a *world-redeemer* (achieve the pinnacle of spiritual power). His father did all he could to lead him to the worldly path but to no avail! He did everything he could to shield Siddhartha from human suffering: poverty, sickness, decrepitude, and death. As the young Siddhartha went on rides outside of his kingly palace, he encountered all of these in the different types of people he met. This led him to seriously doubt that true human happiness and fulfillment could ever be found on the physical plane. Life, he concluded, is inexorably linked with and subject to aging, death, and suffering. Is there any way in which these could be assuaged and overcome? That became his main question and driving force.

Having become aware of the inevitability of bodily pain, deprivation, and death, Gautama could no longer focus his attention upon worldly pleasures and gratifications. So, he left his palace and life, family, riches, and social station, to seek enlightenment. For six years, he led the solitary life of the forest-dweller. First, he looked for the greatest teacher he could find to learn as much as possible about philosophy and raja yoga. Next, he sought the greatest living ascetics and subjected his body to the most difficult and advanced austerities. In the end, he became very weak and fainted. He would have died had his companions not taken care of him. This taught him both the limits and the futility of asceticism. He had experimented with everything that the world and the mind had to offer and had not reached his goal. But he developed the principle of the *Middle Way* between the extremes of asceticism and self-indulgence, of training and working with the body and of training and working with the mind.

During the final phase of his quest, Gautama sought to combine rigorous rational thought with mystical concentration and contemplation, as outlined in raja yoga. One evening, near the town of Patna in Northern India, tired and relaxed, he sat beneath a fig tree which has since popularly be know as the *Bo Tree* (from "Boddhi" or enlightenment). That place was later named the "Immovable Spot" in that Gautama vowed not to rise from it until he had reached illumination. Here he was assailed by all the temptations and allurements of the Devil, *Mara*, to which he resisted just like Jesus did in the desert. Then came the Great Awakening and Siddhartha Gautama emerged the Buddha. The force and bliss of this experience kept the Buddha rooted on this spot for seven days. On the eighth day, he tried to rise but the ecstasy and bliss returned, lasting for a total of 49 days after which he returned to the world.

Mara, the Devil, than appeared to him for one last time with one final and supreme temptation: why not enter final *Nirvana* and forget the world, its delusions and demented beings, why attempt to play the fool before a jury of uncomprehending minds, why try to teach that which can only be experienced and seek to draw the masses away from the passions that still govern them and which they want to satisfy at all costs? The argument contained so much intellectual power and convincing truth that it almost carried the day but, in the end, the Buddha answered, "there will be some who will understand and benefit"! Nearly half a century followed during which the Buddha walked the dusty roads of India.

In the words of Huston Smith, "He founded an order of monks, challenged the deadness of Brahmin society, and accepted in return the resentment, queries, and bewilderment his words provoked. His daily routine was staggering. In addition to training monks, correcting breaches of discipline, and generally directing the affairs of the Order, he maintained an interminable schedule of public preaching and private counseling, advising the perplexed, encouraging the faithful, and comforting the distressed". Cutting across all races, castes, religions, and classes he welcomed all human beings who came to him for guidance and advice.

He died at the age of 80 around the year 480 B.C. after eating some poisoned mushrooms that accidentally ended up on his plate. His parting words to his host, Cunda, who had served him his last and fatal meal were: "Of all the meals I have eaten, two ended up as truly exceptional blessings: the first was the meal that gave me the strength to attain enlightenment under the Bo Tree and the other, my present meal, that opened up the final gates of Nirvana".

Siddhartha's life was driven by the conviction that he had come in this world to perform a *cosmic mission*. Right after his enlightenment, he saw, in his mind's eye, the whole world of humanity moving about *lost*, desperately in need of help and guidance. Hence, he had no choice but to agree with his disciples that he had "been born in this world for the good of the many, the happiness of the seekers, and the evolution of gods and men, out of compassion for the world". The full acceptance of this calling won him both the heart and the mind of India. To many he was known as *Sakyamuni*, the "silent sage", the living embodiment of something that could not be expressed in words or even fathomed by human thinking. He was, unquestionably, a reformer and a rebel Sage that reacted against the decadence and perversion of the Hindu traditions by the religion and clergy of his day.

There are six basic constants that one finds in all religions, indicating that, somehow, these answer the deep, unconscious but structuring needs and aspirations of human beings. These are: *authority, ritual, speculation, tradition, grace* (or God's energies and providence), and *mystery* (always intertwined with mysticism, magic, miracles, and the manifestation of unknown energies and laws). Each seems to be fulfilling important functions in all the religions of man. To Siddhartha, these had become confused and perverted so that the *means* had eaten up and become the *end*. As Prof. Smith aptly put it: "Onto this religious scene, bleak, corrupt, defeatist, and irrelevant, matted with superstition and burdened with irrelevant rituals, Buddha came determined to clear the ground that truth might find purchase and spring again in freshness, truth, and vitality". The result of this was to teach and exemplify a doctrine that was dissociated from these six basic corollaries of religion which, however, in the end, developed its own manifestations of these!

Gautama's approach to religion can be synthesized in the following basic postulates:

- *It was empirical*: for every basic question there was only one final test for truth—*direct personal experience*. A true disciple can only really "know for himself" and nothing else.
- *It was scientific*: direct, personal experience had one basic goal, discovering the cause and effect relationships that order the universe and Life. Hence, the universe, Life, and human experience are based on laws and principles not arbitrariness or luck!
- *It was pragmatic*: it had to always deal with practical *problem solving*, avoiding philosophical and metaphysical speculation. His teachings were "useful tools", "they were like little rafts, helpful for crossing a stream but of no further value once the other side had been reached".
- *It was therapeutic*: like Pasteur, Siddhartha stated "I do not ask you for your opinions or your religion, only what is your suffering?" The existential illness" of the human condition was *suffering* and suffering could be alleviated.
- *It was psychological*: rather than beginning with the outer, material universe or conditions, Buddha always began with man and his problems, his nature and the dynamics of his life in mental and emotional terms.

- *It was democratic*: he rejected the Hindu caste system opening up his Order to all human beings regardless of their religion, race, or sex.
- *It was individualistic*: while Buddha was highly conscious of the social nature of human beings, in the end his essential appeal was always to the individual, individual effort and striving towards enlightenment. "Be ye lamps unto yourselves. Be ye a refuge to yourselves. Betake yourselves to no external judge. Hold fast as a refuge to the Truth . . . work out your own salvation with diligence."

The first sermon that Buddha preached also became the axiomatic core of his message and doctrine. His subject was the Four Noble Truths which he had discovered during his ecstasy under the Bo Tree. These constitute the essential axioms of his system, the basic postulates from which every other aspect of his teaching unfolds. These are:

- The fact that Life is *dukkha*, suffering. It is possible to experience pleasure and enjoyment in life but, in the end, "every pleasure is but disguised pain". For the affairs of men and society are yet in the most imperfect state, bordering on chaos and madness. Thus, his first and most basic postulate is that **human life is misery,** that beyond the glitter of joy and pleasure we have darkness and suffering. Here only one condition is really "real" and that is **pain.**

  This manifests itself as: the trauma of birth, the presence of sickness, the morbidity of decrepitude, the phobia of death, and the separation from what one loves. And the conclusion is that the five *skandas* that define human nature are painful—body, sense, ideas, feelings, and consciousness.
- The cause of life's suffering, or pain, is *tanha*, desire. Wanting, desiring something that one cannot have or do is the root of suffering. But there are two kinds of "desires" that Buddha approved of and advocated: that for liberation and that for the welfare of others. "Tanha" is thus the desires that pull us apart from the rest of life, that are selfish, egoistical, and that come from our ego. It consists of all those inclinations that "tend to continue or increase *separateness*, the separate existence of the person" and thus that render us strangers to reality. As the Buddha states, "rare, indeed, is the man who is more concerned that the standard of life as a whole be raised than that his own salary be increased!" Thus, it is the human self, the ego that makes us suffer. Far from being a door to the more abundant life, the ego is the source root of our suffering.
- If the cause of Life's dislocation and suffering is *selfish craving*, then its cure lies in overcoming such craving. Only when we are released from the narrow limits of self-interest into the expanse of the universal Life are we freed from our torments.

■ The Fourth Noble Truth tells us how this cure can be accomplished: we overcome *tanha* and are released from our captivity through the *Eightfold Path* (EP).

Gautama's perspective on life is essentially that of the *psychotherapist*. He begins by observing carefully the patient, makes his diagnosis, and then proceeds to apply a treatment. People are not what they can and should be. There is more conflict and pain and much less self-expression than is possible thus life is "disjointed", not what it could be. This is "dukkha". What causes suffering and disharmony, what is the seat of infection? The drive for personal, selfish *gratification!* Then, comes the prognosis which brings hope: the disease can be cured by overcoming the egoistic drive for separate existence and ego gratification. Finally, we have the prescription, the overcoming of self-seeking through the Eightfold Path (EP) which is the course of treatment, not an external but an internal treatment—*personal training*. Human beings train themselves for all kinds of disciplines, arts, sports, and sciences; so they can also train themselves for the true "art of living".

The Buddha distinguished between two essential ways of living: one *unconscious*, random, and unreflective where the person is pushed and pulled by external circumstances and internal impulses which he called "wandering about". The other is the *conscious*, intentional way of living which he advocated. He basically designed a "road-map" designed to release the individual from selfishness, impulses, and ignorance. By long and patient discipline the EP intends nothing less than remaking the individual into a different being, a person cured from Life's basic disabilities. "Happiness", he stated can be attained when one *seeks and wins* with training! There is also a preliminary condition which is *right association*, interacting with the right types of persons as we are "social animals" and tend to become like those we interact with. "Companioned example" is thus the precondition. The best way to train an elephant is to yoke him to an already trained elephant!

The EP consists of the following sequential steps:

1. **Right knowledge**. Life needs a blue-print, a map that the mind can trust and which explains what a person is living. What is the heart of these convictions? The Four Noble Truths: that suffering is universal, that it is caused by the desire for separate existence and gratification, that it can be cured, and that the cure is the EP!

2. **Right aspiration**. While the first step involved our minds—what is Life's core problem; the second involves our hearts—what do we really want? Here one must be passionately and single-mindedly pursuing *enlightenment*.

3. **Right speech**. Two switches control our lives and character, *language* and *charity* or compassion. Language is a very good barometer to show our level of consciousness and what we want as well as how we intend to achieve it. The value of truth has ontological, not moral value for behind deceit there is always a fear to reveal to others what we really are and want! False witness, idle chatter, abuse and slander are to be avoided not only because they distort the truth but also because they harm others.

4. **Right behavior**. Before improving our behavior, we need to understand it and its hidden springs more objectively. Essentially, this is similar to the Ten Commandments: do not kill, do not steal, do not lie, do not be unchaste, do not eat or dink intoxicants.

5. **Right livelihood**. The way in which we earn our lives, our occupation, is most important. If our work pulls us in the opposite direction of our spiritual progress, it is incompatible with what we are trying to achieve and become. The "means" becomes the "end"! Some of these include: poison-peddler (the allopathic doctor?), slave dealer, prostitute, butcher, alcohol-maker, armaments maker, and tax collectors.

6. **Right effort**. The will is most important and so is doing the best one can in all occasions. The attainment of love and detachment play an important role here. The training of the will is thus crucial.

7. **Right mindfulness**. No teacher gave the mind a greater importance than the Buddha. This can best be described as "all we are is the result of what we have thought. It is our thoughts that make us what we become". To overcome ignorance (which he saw at the root of all sin and evil) we need mental alertness and self-examination. The level of consciousness and being of a person is directly linked with his self-knowledge and self-mastery.

8. **Right absorption**. This involves the psychospiritual techniques we have seen in raja yoga and leads to the same goal. This is what will really raise consciousness and transform the person. Like a camera whose focal length is ill-focused for the object one wishes to photograph, so the mind of men have been ill-focused for the understanding of reality and must be readjusted. Thus, it is spiritual exercises, *askesis* that will bring about this "re-adjustment".

What is truly most important to human liberation cannot possibly be described in human words; it can only *be lived and experienced*! So is *Nirvana* which is how the Buddha called the state of being brought about by true liberation or spiritual enlightenment. Its best intellectual description is that it is a *condition beyond*—beyond the limitations of the mind, thought, feelings, and will. And it is "bliss", an incredible, fabulous, indescribable and total joy and fulfillment. Its best description in Buddhist texts shows that Nirvana is "permanent, stable, imperishable, immovable, ageless, deathless, unborn, and unbecome. It is power, bliss and happiness". Thus Nirvana could be described as being one with God, not a personal God but the Godhead in all of us!

Buddhism historically evolved and divided itself into three main branches: Mahayana, Hinayana or Theravada Buddhism and Zen. Hinayana Buddhism holds that man is an individual, that he creates his own universe and, therefore, his salvation. That the key virtue is wisdom, that religion is a full-time job (hence for monks). Its ideal is the *Arhat* (the perfected disciple who achieves liberation and Nirvana); the Buddha is a fully actualized human being. It rejects metaphysics and ritual; prayer is essentially meditation and it is conservative.

Mahayana Buddhism, on the other hand, holds that Man is a social being, that he is not alone in the universe, that effort is not sufficient for liberation (grace is also fundamental). Here, the key virtue is compassion and religion is relevant to all, also to those who dedicate themselves to a worldly life. The ideal is the *Bodhisattva* (the realized human being who gives up Nirvana and returns to the world to help his fellow pilgrims); the Buddha is a *world-savior*. It elaborates metaphysics, and includes ritual and prayer; and it is liberal.

After Buddhism slipped into Theravada (small raft) and Mahayana (the big raft), Hinayana Buddhism held together as a single unified tradition whereas Mahayana Buddhism continued to splinter and divide, a little bit like Protestantism in the Christian tradition: one branch emphasizes faith, the other the mind and reason; one gives great importance to ritual while the other emphasizes social action and assumes a political flavor. One branch of intuitive Buddhism that is still very alive today and which established its home in Japan is *Zen* (which means meditation that leads to insight) and which focused almost exclusively upon *direct personal experience*.

Amongst the many paradoxes and contradictions of Buddhism (that we also necessarily find in other religions) perhaps the most important one is that this "religion" which did not begin as such and which revolted against authority, ritual, speculation, grace, mystery and a personal God ended up with all of these in great abundance! Another one is that Buddhism which saw the light in India is now spread over the whole of Asia with the exception of India!

According to Heinrich Zimmer, the great student of oriental religions and Buddhism, there is a basic metaphor, a single image that can explain the differences between the two main forms that Buddhism assumed historically. This is the image of the crossing of a *river on a ferryboat*. Thus Buddhism can be graphically represented as "a voyage across the river of life" where the first shore represents the common-sense shore of spiritual ignorance and of the uninitiated to the far-flung bank of true wisdom which brings liberation from this prevailing bondage—that of the genuine spiritual Initiates and Adepts.

The Theravadins will build a little raft for each individual and then start crossing the river. The Mahayanists move down the banks to where a ferryboat is expected and then board it. The boat leaves and starts the crossing. At first the far-distant shore looks unreal, out-of-focus, and unreachable. As it becomes nearer and near the opposite occurs. The other shore becomes more and more real and into focus while the shore whence the boat started becomes less and less real and more and more out-of-focus! The Theravadin boards the shore and leaves the ship, grateful that it has brought him to this wondrous land. He certainly does not carry it on his back or board it to return whence he came! Then, as he moves inland, there will come a time when not only the raft but even the river drop out of sight and become "unreal", a dream-like fantasy of the mind and past. The Mahayana adept, on the other hand, will take the ferry back to tell his fellow humans what lies on the other shore!

As Huston Smith explains, "Before the river has been crossed, the two shores, human and divine, can appear only as distinct from each other, different as life and death, as day and night. But once the crossing has been made and left behind, no such dichotomy remains. The realm of the gods is no distant place; it is where the traveler stands, and if his stance be still in this world, the world itself has become perfected . . . From this new shore we are now in a position to understand the profound intuition that underlies the Bodhisattva's renunciation. He has paused on the brink of Nirvana, resolved to forgo entering the untroubled pool of eternity until the grass itself becomes enlightened . . . It means that he has risen to the point where the distinction between time and eternity has lost its force, having been made by the rational mind but dissolved in the perfect knowledge of the lightening-and-thunder insight that has transcended the pair of opposites. Time and eternity are now two aspects of the same experience-whole two slices of the same unsliceable completeness. The jewel of eternity is in the lotus of birth and death"!

Chapter VI

JUDAISM

Thus far we have looked at, analyzed, and attempted to explain the essential traditions and core features of the Eastern religions that constitute the outer expression of the Eastern spiritual tradition which roots come from Hinduism. With Judaism, we will leave the East behind and enter the West with its living religions and spiritual tradition which roots originate in Egypt. For reasons of space and time, just as we did not consider a number of Eastern religions, such as Shintoism in Japan, so now we will not be able to consider the Sumerian, Egyptian, and Caldeo-Assirian, and Persian traditions. Likewise, we have been forced to eliminate the African, South Pacific, and South, Central, and American traditions again because of lack of time and as they were not truly essential for our central objective.

I am convinced that by concentrating upon the four major Eastern and the three living Western traditions, we will have a wide enough range and a complete enough canvas of religion to draw major conclusions about human nature, human destiny, the human condition, and what men really want, need and aspire to. Perhaps at a later time in other works and with the help of other interested and competent persons, the present qualitative and quantitative gaps could be filled.

Most important in all of this is the ability to extract a *theoretical framework* and a *practical paradigm*, an intellectual perspective and philosophy of life, as well as basic "instruments" and "guidelines" to develop an *art of living* that is in consonance with our level of consciousness and being and the times in which we are living so as to be able to cope with their greatest challenges, dangers and opportunities.

The Jews were, relatively speaking, late comers on the stage of human history. By 3000 B.C. Egypt already had her religion, spiritual tradition and Pyramids (which constitute the heart and core of the Western spiritual tradition) while Sumer and Akad had already developed world empires. The Jews at that time were a tiny band of nomads milling around the upper region of the Arabian Desert. When they finally settled down, the land they occupied, Palestine, was about as small as the present state of Israel: 150 miles in length and about 50 miles across at Jerusalem, something like one sixth of the state of Pennsylvania!

If the distinctive feature of the Jewish people lies neither in their antiquity nor in the proportions of their land and history, what might it be? According to Huston Smith, what lifted the Jews from obscurity to religious greatness was their *search and passion for meaning*! From the very beginning the Jewish quest for meaning was rooted in their understanding of God, the Creator of all and Ultimate Reality. Whatever a person's philosophy is, it must always take the "other" into account! In that he could not have created himself anymore than other human beings could have created themselves and the universe. Hence, humankind and the universe came from "something" *other* than themselves and this was the starting point of the Jewish faith and tradition!

Confronted with the inevitable *other*, the central question then becomes: is this *other* meaningful and rationally comprehensible? Many rational alternatives presented themselves: this *other* could be incomprehensible, chaotic, amoral, or indifferent if not hostile to human beings. The triumph of Jewish thought lies in its refusal to surrender *meaning* for any other alternative. To make sense of this *other* they personified it! The notion of the inanimate, dead, senseless, unconscious matter governed by blind, impersonal, amoral laws emerged much later in human history and is quite foreign to this tradition.

For early man, the sun, the earth, the rain, storms and lightening, the mystery of birth and death were not to be explained in rational and mechanistic terms but in *spiritual terms* that were filled with strong emotions and a final purpose. Today, we might look upon this as a childish "anthropomorphism" when, in fact, it is purely a question of one's level of consciousness and being and of their sensibilities. At that time, reality appeared far more like a *person* than like the rationalistic and mechanistic *machine* of the 18th, 19th, and 20th centuries! Thus, the Jews, like the Greeks, found a much greater depth and mystery (hence "reality") in human persons rather than in anything else. Where the Jews differed from their neighbors was not in conceiving the *other* as personal, but in perceiving this *other"* in a single, supreme, and transcendental creative power.

In Egypt and Mesopotamia, like in India and China, the divine was seen as being *immanent*: the gods were in and of nature! But the God of the Hebrews was not in nature but *transcended* nature. Their mystics claimed that human beings owed their origin to Him even though their physical bodies were mortal. "Gods are ye, the children of the Most High, all of ye" (Ps. 82:6). For the organized Jewish religion, however, human beings were the subordinates, the servants of God and not His equals. And right from the very beginning, the Jews were monotheists. Their central affirmation and axiom stated: "Hear, O Israel, the Lord our God, the Lord is One".

While for the Greeks, the Romans, the Syrians, and most of the Mediterranean people the gods were amoral and indifferent, the God of the Jews was seen, by their Prophets and Sages, as being righteous, good, and loving being ever-concerned with the welfare of His children, provided these *obeyed Him* (or His Commandments). As Prof. Smith incisively put it, "The Jewish view of the Other with which man is confronted is not prosaic, for at its center sits enthroned a Being of unutterable greatness and holiness. It is not chaotic, for it coheres in a divine unity. The reverse of amoral or indifferent, it centers in a God of righteousness and love". Thus, for them, the word "God" meant a being in whom power and value converge, a being who can do what he wants and who wants to do what is good for men and for his Creation!

But, for most people, most of the time, and in most places, things do not go well. There is suffering, misery and tragedy. How are we to explain this in the light of a God who is powerful and good, wise and moral? Essentially, we have three possible answers: either God does not exist, or He does not care or is not powerful . . . or this is not God's doing but Man's! The Bible clearly states "In the beginning God created the heavens and the earth . . . ; God saw everything that he had made and behold it was very good". While aware of the existence and importance of the spiritual dimension, the Jews refused to conceive of the physical dimension of human existence as being illusory, defective, or unimportant!

Thus life on earth, its abundance and pleasures, were good and should be experienced and made available for the greater number of persons. The core assumption behind the Prophets' denunciation of poverty and inequalities were the opposite of the notion that material possessions are bad. They are so *good and important* that everyone, who lives in a righteous way, should enjoy them and they can be considered as the "blessings" and "rewards" of God to his children. Huston Smith concluded: "The basic premise of the Semitic religions is that the material aspects of life are important (hence the strong emphasis of the West on humanitarianism and social service and justice); that matter can participate in the condition of salvation itself (as affirmed in the doctrine of the Resurrection of the Body!); that nature can become host to the divine (the doctrine of the Kingdom of God on Earth, and, later in Christianity, the Incarnation)."

Next to the meaning of God, comes the meaning of Man, what is a human being? And here, of course, there are as many different answers as there are levels of consciousness and being! In their religion, the Jews concluded, at least in part, that man is, essentially, an *animal.* "The sons of men are in their nature but beasts, the fate of the sons of men and the fate of the beasts is one: as this dies, so dies that, they have the same spirit, and man has no superiority over the beasts (Eccles. 3:18-20). This is a radical an interpretation of human nature as any that the 19th century has produced!

Thus, Man is a spiritual being, a son of the Most High but he is also an animal, a biological organism. How can one reconcile these two different and opposed views—the spiritual grandeur and the biological frailty of human beings? The core insights and concepts that enable us to reconcile these opposite views are those of "sin" and "free will" or *choice*! The concept of "sin" here should be understood in its etymological sense (*amartia* in Greek) of "missing the mark" or falling short of one's destiny and objective.

Prof. Huston summarized this in the following words: "What are the ingredients of the most creatively meaningful image of man that mind can conceive? Remove his frailty—as grass, as a sigh, as dust, as they that are crushed before the moth—and the estimate becomes romantic. Remove his grandeur—a little lower than God—and his aspiration declines. Remove sin—his tendency to miss the mark—and the picture grows sentimental. Remove freedom—choose ye the day—and man becomes a puppet. Remove, finally his sonship to God and man becomes estranged, cut loose and adrift on a sea of blind forces for which he is no match".

In most religions with a trans-empirical frame of reference, ultimate Reality, both within and outside of man, is revealed either through rational contemplation or mystical ascent that go beyond the flow of events on earth that we call history—through a transformation and expansion of human consciousness. The Hebrews, however, being very this-world oriented, argued that God can be found within the limitations of the world—of *history*—in events that are unique, particular, and unrepeatable. Hence, for them, history is neither *Maya* nor a circular process of nature: it is the *arena of God's purposive will and activity*! As such, it is most important, real and meaningful. And this for the following reasons as outlined by Huston Smith:

- First, because they were convinced that the context in which life is lived affects life in every way, setting up its problems, delineating its opportunities, and conditioning its fulfillment.
- Second, if contexts are crucial for life so is *group action*—social action—for there are times when it takes group action to change contexts to the needed extent.
- Third, history was important for the Jews because they saw it always as a field of opportunity. God was the ruler of history; nothing, therefore, happened by accident.
- Finally, history was important because its opportunities did not stream forth on an even plateau. Events, all of them important, were nevertheless not of equal importance . . . The uniqueness of events is epitomized in the Hebraic notion (a) of God's direct intervention in history at certain critical points and (b) of a *chosen people* as recipients of his unique challenges.

As there are special people, Saints, Sages, and Prophets who are God's mouthpiece and instruments on earth, so there is a people that has been chosen for a divine mission—the *Jews*. When Abraham responds to God's call and is ready to answer it at whatever cost (e.g. the sacrifice of his only son, Isaac), he ceases to be anonymous and becomes the first of the Hebrew, the "seed of the chosen people". Judaism sets history as being both important and subject to improvement.

Man is a historical being but because he has misused his freedom, he has corrupted history and denied himself the full range of the expression of his potentialities! Thus history is in tension between divine potentialities and man's corruption of them and there is a profound disharmony or dichotomy between God's will and the existing social order. This is how Judaism, more so than any other religion, laid the groundwork for social protest and reforms. As things are not the way they should be, change is needed, and revolution is to be expected!

For Judaism, man is a *social animal;* he cannot become human and remain at the level of the beasts. Hence both wisdom and discipline are needed to keep his relationships from breaking down. The Hebrew's formulation of these "wise restraints that keep men healthy and free" is to be found in her Law which contains both ritualistic and ethical prescriptions. There are no less than 613 commandments in the Old Testament that regulate human behavior. Their essence and root are to be found in the Ten Commandments that made its greatest impact upon the world. Taken over by both Christianity and Islam, these constitute the moral foundation of more than half the world's present population.

In human life, there are four dangers that can cause unlimited trouble if they get out of hand and which do not exist in the animal world which is governed by instincts. These are: force, wealth, sex, and the spoken word. It is these that the Ten Commandments seek to keep in check and harmony. Western civilization is rooted in the double conviction that: the future of any people depends largely on the justice of their social order and that individuals are responsible for the condition of their society as well as for the affairs of their personal lives. This was the core message of the Hebrew Prophets. While the earlier Prophets challenged essentially individuals, later Prophets challenged the structure and establishment of existing societies.

In essence, the Prophetic insight was that the prerequisite for political stability is always *social justice* and that social injustice breeds its own demise for such was the will of the Lord! This led to the conviction that every man simply by virtue of the fact that he is human, that he is a child of God, *has rights that even kings and armies cannot erase!* Prophets exist and come upon the stage of history as a strange, elemental and explosive force. As Huston Smith puts it, "They live in a vaster world than those about them, a world in which pomp and ceremony, wealth and splendor, count for nothing, where kings seem small and the power of the mighty is nothing compared to *purity, justice,* and *mercy*". And this, I might add, is true not only of the Hebrew Prophets but of the Saints, Sages, and spiritually awakened Persons of every race and religion.

Israel and Judah were very small tribes compared to the aggressive power of Syria, Assyria, Egypt, and Babylon but these were perceived by the Prophets as the "instruments of God" to punish a wayward child that no longer obeyed his father! Thus the persecutions and sufferings of the Jews were perceived first as a "wake-up call" to honor their Covenant with God or as a "punishment" for not doing so. Later, however, suffering was redefined from a *punishing* to a *learning* experience and as a *redemptive experience* for the world. What the Jews learned from their captivity (Egypt and Babylon), in the words of Prof. Smith, was "Through their suffering God was burning indelibly into the hearts of the Jews a passion for freedom and justice, counting on these to spread from them to all mankind".

In Judaism there is a firm conviction that all of life down to the smallest detail can be made holy and to conform to God's will. This is what *piety* meant to them. It is thus piety that prepares the way for the coming of God's kingdom on earth, the time when everything will be redeemed and sanctified so that the will of God will be made manifest in all creation. Thus, throughout Judaism we find a double theme: enjoy the pleasures of life and increase this joy by sharing it with God. This is how Jewish law sanctions all the good things of life—eating, sex, marriage, children, nature, and sports—while elevating them to holiness. Hence, it teaches human beings how they should approach and deal with almost everything. The sanctity of all things should and can be preserved through *tradition.* As Huston Smith puts it, "Without attention, man's sense of wonder and the holy will stir occasionally, but to become a steady flame they must be deliberately fed."

One of the ways in which this can be accomplished is to be steeped in *history that shows God's acts of providence and mercy in every generation!* Against those that would forget the past and its memories, Judaism sees it as one of the most priceless treasures! Judaism is thus one of the most *historically minded religions,* finding holiness and history to be inseparable. The key is thus to learn how to "live within time the life of eternity". The basic manual for doing so and hallowing the whole of life is the first five books of the Bible, the Torah which, for the Jews, is like a "tree of Life to those who can grasp it"!

Unlike other Western religions, Judaism never promulgated an official doctrine or creed that one must adhere to in order to be considered a Jew. It is observance and ritual that they emphasized and demanded, together with the ethic of the Ten Commandments. In spite of their trials and tribulations, they always emphasized and underscored *God's great goodness to man,* which they then sought to justify and explain in terms of the possible *meaning* and *significance* of human events. The Old Testament, as the New, is steeped in *revelation,* which is what the Prophets brought that enabled people to make sense of their experiences. Revelation means awareness, disclosure, understanding, understanding of God and of His will for man in particular. And for the Jews, unlike the Greeks or the Hindus, God revealed himself through what *He did* and not through words or ideas!

For the Hebrews, God did two things that really stand out: he enabled them to survive and he brought them out of captivity in Egypt! As Huston Smith explained: "The Exodus, that incredible incident in which God liberated an unorganized, enslaved people from the mightiest power of the age, was not only the event that launched the Jews as a nation. It was also the first clear act by which God made known to the Jews the fullness of His nature". Hence, God was first and foremost a God of *power,* with enough power to outdo the mightiest empire, but he was equally a God of *goodness* and *love.* Though this might be less transparent to others, it was evident to the Jews who were the immediate beneficiary of these characteristics. "Happy art Thou, O Israel; who is like unto thee, a people saved by Yahweh?" (Deut. 33:29).

Moreover, the Jews had done nothing to deserve this and so it was a pure act of love and grace. Besides God's power and love, the Exodus also clearly showed that God was interested in human beings, their doings and lives. Hence he was concerned with *history* and was quite different from the gods that were working primarily through the *forces of nature.* Thus, for the Jews, it was unthinkable that a God that had been so good to His people in the beginning would ever desert them and cease to care for them in their history and becoming. To explain their sufferings and persecutions, the Jews developed the notion of a *Covenant* with God, of a contract whereby God would take care of them if they obeyed God and His Commandments. If they did not they would be chastised and punished. This is what we found in the Abraham epic. Abraham remained faithful to God and obeyed His will even to the point of being ready to sacrifice his only son thus God rewarded him by giving him a good land (hence life) and innumerous descendants.

Why would this "revelation" or disclosure be made to the Jews and not to other people? Their own answer has been because *we were chosen!* This messianic conclusion, however, was also reached by many other people and religions, the Japanese, who thought they were the "children of the Sun", the French, who were convinced that they has been chosen to promulgate liberty, equality, and fraternity, and the Christians who argued that they had been given the one and only final revelation and salvation. The Jewish doctrine of election began in a conventional mode but their Prophets emphasized that they were chosen as the recipients of special privileges so that they serve and suffer the ordeals necessary for the salvation of the world.

Finally, the acceptance of the lofty demands of the Torah also opened them to penalties and retribution if they did not live it! Prof. Smith concludes: "The fact that He singled them for a role of special partnership in the redemption of the world is still an indication that He held them in special regard and even love . . . Israel was brought into being as a nation by an extraordinary occurrence in which a nondescript group of slaves broke the bonds of the mightiest power on earth and were lifted to the status of a free and self-respecting people". The prophetic protest against social injustice was its consequence and one that the modern state of Israel should pay close attention to.

As Huston Smith concludes: "Nothing does more to explain the extraordinary response the Jews made to their diverse and severe challenges that have befallen them than the conviction that God loved them uniquely and was counting on them to make His will known and bring healing to the nations". Is this true? This is a point that no one can establish objectively. I would argue that any person who reaches the *soul-level*, who establishes a living connection between the conscious and the superconscious will have a similar experience: God loves them and has chosen them for a special mission—to reveal His love and will to all people. The famous Jewish saying, "You are my servant, Israel, in whom I will be glorified" could thus be applied to any person, of any race and religion, who has achieved genuine *spiritual consciousness* that makes him aware of the love and will of God!

Obviously, as in every other religion, there are great individual differences and interpretations of the same insight and idea—which to me represent *different levels of consciousness and being*. So also in Judaism we find the whole range that goes from extreme fundamentalism to ultra-liberalism and secularism. Jewish culture, which represents a *total way of life* (including folkways, art forms, food specialties, styles of humor and philosophy) has crystallized around three basic aspects: language, lore, and an affinity for a land, Israel. As Huston Smith incisively concluded, "The Torah is followed by the Talmud, a vast compendium of law, commentary, history, and folklore which is the basis of post Biblical Judaism. This in turn is supplemented by the *Misdrashim*, an almost equal collection of legend, exegesis, and homily which began to develop before the Biblical canon was fixed and was not completed until the late Middle Ages. The whole provides an inexhaustible mine for scholarship, anecdote, and general cultural enrichment."

A final note here is that if it is true that the quintessential interest and characteristic of the Hebrew tradition is the *quest for meaning*, for making rational sense out of the myriad of human experiences that make up the *condition humaine*, then it is easy to deduce that another great Prophet appeared, in the 20th century, in that tradition: Viktor Frankel, the Viennese psychiatrist who wrote a most important book in a concentration camp, *Man's search for Meaning* and who developed a school of psychotherapy known as *Logotherapy*. Essentially, Frankel argued, a human being will be able to face any human situation and not break down provided he continues to perceive some *meaning and purpose in it*!

As a medical doctor at Auschwitz Frankel had noticed that some people died for no organic cause while others continued on living. Seeking an explanation for this strange paradox, he concluded that those that survived still perceived some meaning and purpose in their happenings while the ones that died no longer did. This is how Logotherapy was born, which represents the quintessence of the Hebrew tradition in the modern world if we accept the basic assumption that what always distinguished Jews from others was a *quest and passion for meaning*.

In dealing with religion, with any religion, it is most important to draw a sharp distinction between what it *stands for*, it's idealistic formulation and revelation, and how it is *lived and put into practice*. All great world religions are valid and contain great universal ideals but these are not always interpreted and lived in the same way. Here, another truly essential factor which we must understand and take into account is *the level of consciousness and being* of those who profess and live a given religion. All paradoxes, contradictions, and oppositions can be explained by this truly fundamental insight which I have sought to articulate in my image of "Man the skyscraper" and of the analogy of the "vertical axis of consciousness". Most excesses, abuses, and perversions of religion have come from people on a low level of consciousness and being who have instrumentalized and distorted what their tradition taught and who used its teachings and precepts for separation rather than union, for hatred rather than love, and for death rather than for life—hence for self rather than for Self.

Chapter VII

CHRISTIANITY

In my opinion, it is very important to be able to distinguish clearly and to draw a sharp distinction between "Christianity" and the "Christian denominations": Eastern Orthodoxy, Roman Catholicism, and Protestantism that make up the contemporary Christian religion. While this may sound like an "unusual" or "radical proposition", it really is not. The spiritual tradition always made that distinction and St. Augustine expressed it, clearly and explicitly, when he stated that "Christianity always existed and was not created or did not come into being with the birth and the teachings of Jesus of Nazareth". Christianity, whose central goal has always been to lead its practitioners to become fully actualized and "Christed" Human Beings," has indeed always existed and was always the conscious and overt or unconscious and covert goal of human life!

As such, "Christianity" is really the historical and external manifestation of the "Holy Wisdom", the *Philosophia Perennis*, the essential knowledge and practice, to realize the "Christian state or level of consciousness and being". Jesus of Nazareth embodied and lived this realization and offered to all those to whom this appealed and who wanted to follow Him so as to also realize this sublime achievement. He did not create another religion or another interpretation of the Jewish religion, rather He took the ancient Initiation with all of its symbols and allegories and incarnated it, *lived it*, so that it could be given to the world, to the many, rather than reserving it for the few, the few "elect" who had been especially trained and prepared for it. It is only later, a few centuries later, that Christianity became a religion which then fragmented into different branches with several sprouts.

Following the outline and the core insights suggested by Huston Smith, let me begin with the "Christian denominations" and, in the end, seek to bring these together in the heart of Christianity . . . as Christianity is the "heart" of all religions and wisdom traditions. Prof. Smith begins by saying that Christianity is basically a *historical* religion, grounded more in concrete events and actual historical happenings rather than in universal principles. My position, of course, is that it is *both* but that what we know as Christianity today is essentially the former. The most important of these "historical happenings" are, as Prof. Smith stated, "The life of a little-known Jewish carpenter who, as has often been pointed out, was born in a stable, died at the age of thirty-three as a criminal rather than a hero, never traveled more than 90 miles from his birthplace, owned nothing, attended no college, marshaled no army, and instead of producing books did his only writing in the sand! Nevertheless . . . his birthday is kept across the world and his death-day sets a gallows against every skyline". Who and what was He?

This is a truly fundamental question that countless people have asked themselves and that Jesus Himself asked his disciples, Peter in particular, to answer. As such, it is a question that each one of us will have to ask at some point in our human and spiritual evolution. The problem here is that "only like can know like", that the higher may know and understand the lower but not vice-versa! In ultimate analysis, only the divine can know the Divine . . . and that the very same thing or event can be perceived, defined, and reacted to in very different and even opposite ways! When we try to pin down His biographical details, we are immediately struck at how scarce and vague these are. We do know that He was born in Palestine, probably around 4 B.C. He grew up in or around Nazareth. He was baptized by John, a recognized Prophet who was proclaiming that God's Judgment was at hand. He had a teaching-healing career that lasted about three years and which took place in Galilee.

He incurred the hostility of some of his own as well as the suspicion of the Romans even though He went about "doing good", bringing healing and enlightenment to countless people. John Knox argued that the Gospels did not succeed in fully revealing Who Jesus was just as they were unable to conceal Him. Thus he concluded, "Whatever may be lacking in our picture of Jesus, we know more than enough to characterize Him as a person of strange and incomparable greatness". What led so many people to conclude that He was divine? The answer can come in three basic parts: what He did, what He said, and what He was. Beginning with the first, it is undeniable that He did much good wherever He went. Though He performed many "miracles", He never used them as a means to convert or to convince others. Almost all of His extraordinary deeds were performed quietly, apart from the crowds, and as a demonstration of the power of *faith* which, potentially, *every person also had*. Wherever He went, he sought to bring hope, healing, faith, and goodness in people so that they, in turn, concluded that "God is pure Love or Goodness"!

The great Jewish scholar Klausner stated, "If you take the teachings of Jesus separately, you can find every one of them paralleled in either the Old Testament or its commentary, the Talmud. If, on the other hand, you take them as a whole, they have an urgency, an ardent vivid quality, an abandon, and above all a complete absence of second-rate material that makes them refreshingly new". In other words, it is not so much **what** He said as **how** He said it, the power and authority He put into His words that really stood out. As Prof. Smith put it, "The language of Jesus is a fascinating study in itself, quite apart from its content . . . If simplicity, concentration, and the sense of what is *vital* are marks of great religious literature, these qualities alone would make Jesus' words immortal. But this is just the beginning. They carry an extravagance of which wise men, mindful of their capacity for balanced judgment, are incapable."

And, he concluded, "Indeed, their passionate quality has led one poet to coin a special word for Jesus' language, calling it "gigantesque". If your hand offends you, cut it off. If your eye stands between you and the best, gouge it out. Jesus is always talking about camels going through needles' eyes, of men who fastidiously strain the gnats from their drink while oblivious of the camels bumping down their gullets. His characters go around with timbers protruding from their eyes looking for tiny specks in the eyes of their neighbors. He talks of people whose outer lives are stately as mausoleums while their inner lives stink as of bodies in putrefaction. This is not rhetorical technique skillfully added for effect. The language is part of the Man Himself, stemming from the urgency and passion of His driving conviction".

As for what He said, quantitatively, it does not amount to very much, but the quality and pointedness of what He said is truly remarkable in that in very few words He really hit the "essentials" and the fundamental cosmic Laws of life. All the words of Jesus recorded in the New Testament could be spoken out in less than two hours and yet they are the most repeated words in the world! A good practical example is: "Love your neighbor as yourself". "Whatsoever ye would that men should do unto you, do ye also unto them". "Come unto me, all ye that labor and are heavy laden, and I will give you rest". "Ye shall know the truth and the truth shall make you free". Most of the time, he told stories, parables, with multiple meanings, implications and applications depending upon one's level of consciousness and being (the buried treasure, the sowers, the merchants and the pearl of great value, the good Samaritan, the young man who blew his entire inheritance on a great binge, etc.). People who heard these parables for the first time generally responded by saying "never spake man thus"!

As Huston Smith summarized it: "We are told that we are not to resist evil; that we are to turn the other cheek; and to love our enemies and bless them that curse us. The world assumes that friends are to be loved and enemies hated. That the sun rises on the just and the unjust alike . . . . And the world resents this, feeling that the sun ought to rise only on the just . . . It is offended when the wicked go unpunished, and would prefer seeing them living under perpetual clouds . . . We are told that the publican and the harlot go into heaven before many who are outwardly righteous, whereas the world, wrapped in conventions and conformity assumes that it is safest to follow the crowd . . . . We are told to be as carefree as birds of the air and the lilies of the field while the world assumes that we should take care to build our security". Essentially, He was trying to move us from the *horizontal* to the *vertical* dimension, from the world of duality to the world of unity and to the reconciliation of polarities and opposites.

The quintessence of what He was trying to tell us is truly simple but fundamental. It is: *God's overwhelming love for man* and *the need for man to receive this love and to let it flow out and circulate in the world.* Prof. Smith concludes: "God had been unswerving in His loving kindness and stubborn love. Time after time, as in the story of the shepherd who risked ninety-nine sheep to go after one that had gone astray, Jesus tries to convey *God's absolute love for every single one of His children.* To perceive this love, nay to feel it to the very marrow, was to respond in the only way possible, in profound and total gratitude for the wonders of God's grace." Every human being, every person, for Jesus, has *infinite worth and value* precisely because he is God's Child, the heir of all the treasures and potentialities of both the universe and of divinity! Essentially, Jesus brought three priceless treasures: *The Kingdom of Heaven* (the awakening of spiritual consciousness), *the Powers of the Holy Spirit* (all the psychic and parapsychological powers but used only to do God's Will) and *a living model and archetype* of what a human being truly is and can become!

When we come to what He *was*, we are confronted with the insurmountable barrier that "only like can know like" and thus that only God can know God! We must be content with translating, in terms of our own level of consciousness and being, our perception and understanding of what He was. The most impressive thing about the teachings of Jesus is not what He taught but how He *lived* what He said! As Huston Smith puts it: "His entire life was one of complete humility, self-giving and love which sought not His own. The supreme evidence of His humility . . . is that it is impossible to discover precisely what Jesus thought of Himself! He was not concerned that men should know what He was. His concern was for people to know God and His Will for their lives . . . He thought infinitely less of Himself than He did of God. It is impossible to read what Jesus said about selflessness without sensing at once how free He was of pride. The same is true of His observations on sincerity—they could not have been uttered by anyone tinctured by deceit. Truth was to Him as the air, falsity as suffocating as a tomb."

Above all Jesus hated hypocrisy because it created many outer and inner disharmonies and cut a person off from himself and from Reality. Hypocrisy hid a man from himself and precluded him from truly relating to others, as well as to himself, and thus making *exchanges* that are so essential for life and evolution. As Prof. Smith aptly penned it, "In the end, especially when He laid down his life for His friends, it seemed to those who knew Him best that here was a man in whom *the human had disappeared completely,* leaving His life so *completely under the Will of God* that it became perfectly transparent to that Will. It came to the point where they felt that as they looked at Jesus they were looking at the way God would be if He were to assumed human form." This is what led the Disciples to say, "We beheld His glory, the glory of the only begotten Son of the Father, full of grace and truth."

Jesus ended His short ministry by being crucified. This might well have been the tragic end of His story as it was for many visionaries who achieved great status and popularity while alive but who were quickly forgotten once they died! As He Himself had foretold it, three days later, He Resurrected and, within a few days, His disciples were preaching the gospel of Christ, the risen Lord. Mary of Magdala had gone to His Tomb and found it empty, the stone that closed it having been rolled away. Thereafter, Jesus appeared to her and sporadically to a few of His disciples. It was the belief in His *Resurrection* that gave impetus for the rise of the Apostolic Church and the development of the Christology that underpinned it. As Huston Smith pointed out, "it was the news that Christ had risen and with it the implication that those who believed in Him could, like Him and with Him, *triumph over sin and death to new life*" that made His message irresistible and that became the cornerstone of the Christian faith.

His Resurrection also clearly pointed out to a most crucial union: that of *goodness with power!* In the life of Jesus, the disciples had found *essential goodness incarnated*, in His Resurrection, they found the manifestation of *supreme power!* Again, as Huston Smith saw it, "If Golgotha's cross had been the end, the goodness of Christ embodied would have been tragically beautiful, but how insignificant? A fragile blossom afloat on a torrent, soon to be dashed—how relevant is goodness if it has no purchase on reality, no power at its disposal? The Resurrection completely reversed the cosmic status in which goodness had been left by the crucifixion. Instead of being pitiful it was victorious, triumphant over everything, even the end of all ends—*death itself*"!

Thus, if Christ's Life and Death had convinced the disciples of God's *Love*, His Resurrection convinced them of God's *Power*, demonstrating conclusively that the worst that the dark powers and evil men can do (torture and crucified the One that loved them most) and even that the seemingly inexorable and unfeeling laws of nature (death) cannot block God's work and purpose. The disciples and the first Christians were thus convinced that no essential harm could ever befall them as they stood sustained by Christ's Power forever. As Prof. Smith incisively put it, "Back to the original Christians. Whether or not Jesus' body actually rose from the grave, no one can doubt that His Spirit jumped dramatically to life, transforming a dozen or so disconsolate followers of a slain and discredited leader into one of the most creative groups in human history . . . This was the Good News that snapped Western history like a dry twig into B.C. and A.D. and left its impact throughout the Christian Church . . ."

"Was it Jesus' ethical teachings—the Golden Rule, the Sermon on the Mount, loving one's enemies? Not at all . . . it was neither Jesus' ethical precepts nor even the phenomenal way in which His Life had exemplified them. It was something quite different . . . It was the enterprise of Life itself (a philosophy and an art of living as I would call them) . . . They seemed to have found the secret of **living**. They evidenced a tranquility, simplicity, and cheerfulness that their hearers had nowhere else encountered. Here were people who seemed to be making a success of the greatest enterprise of all, the enterprise of Life itself." Two fundamental qualities stood out from the early Christians' lives: *Love* that leads to true self-expression and growth and genuine *Brotherhood* or equality! The earliest observations, from outsiders, about Christians were "see how they love each other" for to them, the conventional barriers of race, religion, and status were nothing (For in Christ there is neither Jew nor Gentile, Greek or barbarian, rich or poor)."

The second fundamental quality was *joy!* Before His Crucifixion, Jesus told His disciples, "My joy I leave with you". Outsiders found this baffling and unbelievable, something literally, "out of this world"! The scattered Christians were not numerous, wealthy, or powerful. They faced more adversity and persecution that most people have ever faced and yet, they had an *inner peace, a joy, and a radiance* that defy adequate description, a "joy unspeakable and full of glory" as it has been described. What produced this love, peace, joy, and goodness, qualities that are universally coveted but very rarely achieved? According to the New Testament it was the removal of three intolerable and universal burdens that face all human beings: *the fear of death, the torment of guilt,* and a *release from the constricting confines of the ego*! The most profound and incisive answer was given by Paul when he declared, "I live, yet not I but Christ in me". Thus the vicious circle of *ego-ism*, the rule of the human self, was broken, leaving love and life able to flow freely in those who had realized this state of consciousness.

The only power that can effectively bring about the above described transformations is *genuine love*. There is here and interesting outer/inner analogy. In the 20th century, physicists discovered and unlocked the power of the atom which contains a miniature solar system with the power of the sun itself (nuclear fission). Mystics and spiritually awakened persons have always known experientially that locked up at the very center of a human being lays the "treasure of treasures" the love and power of God which can also be released by the progressive development and expression of human love. What the early Christians discovered was precisely the *love of God* which they could feel and experience. They became convinced that Jesus was God as God had fully and consciously *incarnated in Him* and many did, in fact, experience the power of His Love . . . which melted down the barriers of *fear, guilt, and ego!*

The first Christians who preached the Good News did not feel alone, they were convinced that their Leader was in their midst as a living, energizing Power.

They remembered Him saying, "Wherever two or three of you are gathered in My Name, there I am in the midst of them". Mindful of what Paul had stated, "For as the body is one and hath many members and all are the members of the same body, whereas they are many, yet they are one body as is Christ". The Church was the mystical body of Christ. Christ was the Head, the Holy Spirit its soul, and individual Christians, the cells of the same body, first few in number but then more as the body matured. To become part of that body, you had to believe in Him, apply His teachings, and follow His living example. But there is the visible Church and also the invisible Church, the Church militant on earth and the Church triumphant in Heaven, to which the earthly church is but one door!

For the early Christians as for the Orthodox Church later, it was not the mind that came first in responding to Christ, it was *experience* that came first—the experience of living in the actual presence of God. As Prof. Smith explained, "Once the Christian experience had occurred, it was only a matter of time until the mind would seek to interpret this experience and Christian theology was born. From then on the Church would be mind as well as heart." Within Christianity there was always a tension and an opposite pulling between the ethical teachings of Jesus and the more mystical arguments of Paul, between the "religion of Jesus" and the "religion about Jesus", between the human Jesus and the cosmic Christ. A child growing up has two fundamental questions: *how should I behave?* And *what are the limits of toleration of my parents beyond which I will be rejected?*

The idea of God's love was not new and could be found in all authentic religion, but in Christ's presence it ceased to be an idea to become a *living reality*. The doctrine of the Incarnation affirms that in Christ God assumed a human body, that Christ was God-Man, simultaneously fully God and fully Man. As Prof. Smith explained, "In saying that Jesus was God, one thing the Church was saying is that His Life provides the perfect model by which men may order their lives" which became the *imitatio Christi!* What was truly astonishing and revolutionary here was not that God might walk the earth in human form, but that *He would voluntarily suffer for Man's sake!* Christ therefore was God's mirror: to know what God is *look at Christ.*"

In looking at the doctrine of the Atonement, we find that its root is *reconciliation*, re-uniting one's self with God through the part of God that was within one's self, in the depths of one's being and in the heights of one's consciousness. In Christ, as Paul states, God was reconciling the world unto Himself. The estrangement between God and Man is the work of "sin" and "sin" means missing (Greek *amartia*) one's target or objective. The early Christian had sins removed by the Presence and Energies of the Christ and thus their alienation from God was also removed. Then came the concept of the Trinity which is and remains a profound mystery with many levels of interpretations depending upon one's level of consciousness and being. God and Man have three structural levels (the body, the soul, and the spirit) and three functional levels (Wisdom, Love, and Life); thus man confronts God in three basic ways: *in the mysteries of Nature, in the historical Person of Christ,* and *in the depths of his own heart.* While distinct these are equally God! God is Love but Love can only be generated and circulated by Persons!

From its essential, original trunk, Christianity historically splintered and manifested into three main branches: Eastern Orthodoxy linked with John, Roman Catholicism linked with Peter, and Protestantism linked with Paul. Another metaphor would be to say that it has a "spirit, a soul, and a body" which are quite different from each other but that complement and complete each other. Thus the very same phenomenon, process, or occurrence can be perceived, interpreted, and reacted to in very different ways depending on one's "vertical axis" (level of consciousness and being or evolution) and "horizontal axis" (personal experiences, values, and "points of reference").

This is exactly what happened to Christianity, as well as to any other religion, as it moved forward in time and articulated itself in the world. Through what I call the perspective of the "human sky-scraper", we can rationally understand most paradoxes and contradictions and learn how to live with different ways of perceiving and articulating anything—in other words, we can "agree to disagree" and be tolerant of those who do not see things the way we do. Babies, children, adolescents, young adults, mature adults, and older person simply do not see and respond to things in the same way! It is interesting to note that ethnicity, culture, climate and regional history have a major impact upon how a religion is going to be perceived, interpreted, and lived.

In the words of Huston Smith: "When we turn from early Christianity to Christendom today, we find the Church divided into three great branches. Roman Catholicism focuses in the Vatican, in Rome, and spreads from there, being dominant, on the whole, through central and southern Europe, Ireland and South America. Protestantism dominates northern Europe, England, Scotland, and North America. The third great division, Eastern Orthodoxy, has major influence in Greece, the Slavic countries and the U.S.S.R.". Historically, three major "turning points" occurred: the first in the 4th Century when Christianity, from being a persecuted sect became the dominant religion of the Roman Empire, and when the truly original spiritual, initiatory or esoteric aspects began to diminish and go "underground" as large numbers of people, many of whom were far from being spiritually ready, were brought into its fold.

The second "turning point" occurred in the 12th Century when the East, focused on *direct personal experience,* and the West, focused on *reason, rationalization,* and *organization,* broke away giving rise to Eastern Orthodoxy and Western Roman Catholicism. The third and final "splintering" occurred in the 16th Century with the Protestant Reformation as the process of secularization and rationalization continued on its path in human evolution. I believe that we are now (end of the 20th and beginning of the 21st Centuries) in the process of bringing about yet a fourth transformation, *the birth of spiritual science*, linked with the development of the scientific method and the articulation of Science as the royal path to Truth and Reality, that might bring together the three major branches, as well as the other world religions, in a higher and more practical *synthesis* and *application*. I see this as the reunion of the "body, soul, and spirit of religion", of the "letter with the spirit", of its exoteric, outer, non-mystical aspects with its esoteric, inner, and mystical aspects—the "religion of the masses" and the "religion of the Saints and Sages"—which corresponds to our present level of consciousness and being and evolution!

As Huston Smith concluded: "Roman Catholicism holds that the Trinity actually dwells in every Christian soul, but its presence is not normally felt (as It dwells at the superconscious level). By a life of prayer and penance it is possible to dispose oneself for a special gift whereby the Trinity discloses Its presence (brings It from the superconscious into the conscious) and the seeker is lifted to a state of *mystical ecstasy*. But as man has no right to such states, they being wholly in the nature of free gifts of grace, the Roman Church neither urges nor discourages the mystical more actively. The Eastern Church has encouraged the mystical life more actively. From early times when the deserts near Antioch and Alexandria were filled with hermits seeking illumination, the entire mystical enterprise has occupied a more prominent place in her life.

As the supernatural world intersects and impregnates the world of sense and reason throughout, it should be a part of Christian life in general to develop the capacity to experience directly the glories and God's Presence . . . . Mysticism (here) is a practical program even for laymen. The aim of every life should be *union with God*, actual *deification* to the point of sharing the Divine Life. As our destiny is to enter creatively into the Life of the Trinity, the love that circulates incessantly among Father, Son, and Holy Spirit, movement toward this goal should be a part of every Christian life."

In essence, the Roman Catholic Tradition is grounded in the twin principles of "The Church as the supreme Teaching Authority" and of "The Church as the Sacramental Channel" just as the Protestant Tradition is anchored upon the twin principles of "Justification by Faith" and of "Radical Monotheism". In a sense they are both opposed and complementary, touching and bringing out different facts and aspects of human nature and of the human condition. It is only in a higher level of consciousness and being and through the mystical or spiritual tradition that these can be properly understood, evaluated, and reconciled.

To avoid chaos and confusion and to structure their activities on earth, people need Authority and leaders that interpret and uphold this Authority. The Catholic tradition postulates that God came on earth in the person of Jesus Christ to teach people how to live in order to achieve Salvation. If His Teachings really hold the door to "Salvation" then a "vehicle" is needed to teach, perpetuate, and interpret these teachings. The Bible is the *physical body* of these Teachings which need to be properly adapted and interpreted, and that vehicle, or "soul", is the "Church". The Sacraments are the channels through which *grace*, the higher energies of God, can be conveyed to people so that they will be able to accomplish what they came to do in this world. For it is one thing to be able to *know what we must do* and quite another to actually *be able to do it!* As Prof. Smith aptly puts it, "The Church helps with both problems. It points the way we should live and it also supplies us with the power to live in this way".

Huston Smith concludes, "Christ called His followers to live lives far above the average in charity and service . . . . Without help such a life is impossible. For the life to which Christ called men is supernatural in the exact sense of being contrary to the pull of man's natural instincts. By his own efforts man can no more live above his nature than an elephant can live a life of reason. Help, therefore, is obviously necessary. The Church, as God's representative on earth, is the Agency to provide it, and the Sacraments are the means for doing so."

For the Protestant tradition, Man is saved by Faith alone and not by his own efforts, good and heroic as these may be. Faith, however, is a personal phenomenon; it is a direct *personal* experience which is unique to the individual and which only God can confer. As Prof. Smith incisively puts it, "Faith is the response by which God, heretofore a postulate of philosophers and theologians, becomes God to me, *my God*. This is the meaning of Luther's statement that "Everyone must do his own believing as he will have to do his own dying". And this led to the Protestant primacy of the *individual conscience* of each person and of his *personal salvation*.

As for "Radical Monotheism", or the "Protestant Principle" as some called it, it warns us about absolutizing what is relative or, in theological terms, it rings a strong bell about *idolatry*. As Prof. Smith explains, "Man's allegiance belongs to God and to God alone. God, however, is beyond nature and history. He is removed from these, but He cannot be equated with either or any of their parts, for while the world is emphatically finite, God is infinite . . . While the secular world proceeded to absolutize the state or the self of man's intellect, Christians fell to absolutizing dogmas, Sacraments, the Church, the Bible, or even personal experience. To think that Protestantism devalues these or doubts that God is involved in them is to seriously misjudge its stance. But it does determinedly insist that none of them is God . . . As long as each points beyond itself to God, it is invaluable. But let any claim man's absolute or unreserved allegiance—which is to say to usurp God's place—and it becomes diabolical"!

The above are some of the main distinctions between the three basic branches of Christianity which, unfortunately, have fought each other in very bloody and unchristian ways for centuries, when, in fact, from the standpoint of a higher level of consciousness and being, they *complement* each other. At this point in my evolution as see them as the "spirit, the soul, and the body" of the same Being, the Mystical Body of Christ which, at the end of time, will include every single human being with no exception! For the time being, we must "agree to disagree", we must realize that we are not all functioning on the same level of consciousness, being, and evolution; hence, that we do not perceive and define the same thing in the same way . . . and that we have the right to our own perceptions and conclusions; not only, if we want to make true human and spiritual progress we must be *true to ourselves* . . . whatever the effort and cost involved!

Chapter VIII

ISLAM

First, it is important to clarify one point concerning the last of the great Western World Religions, that of its name. Sometimes, Islam is called "Mohammedanism", which would be both offensive to the Muslims and inaccurate. "Islam" means "surrender to God's Will" and Mohammed was the Prophet who received that revelation from God through the Archangel Gabriel and who embodied it in the Koran; he certainly did not and could not have created it and articulated it himself! He was merely its "channel" or "vehicle", great a man that he was. The Koran names God *Allah* which is made up two particles, "Al", meaning "The" and "Illah" which means "God". Allah thus means "The God" or better the only or One, true God. Allah created the world and then created the first Man, Adam (which Islam shares with Judaism and Christianity). The descendants of Adam led to Noah who had a son, Shem, which is the root of the word "Semite" which means descendent of Shem, so the Arabs consider themselves a Semitic people. It was the complete submission of Abraham to God's Will (being willing to sacrifice his only son, the greatest treasure he had, and described in the Koran by the verb *aslama)* that appears to have given Islam its name (complete surrender to God's Will).

Abraham married Sarah but had no son and so Abraham married Hagar who gave him a son, Ishmael. At that point, Sarah also bore him a son, Isaac and demanded that Hagar and Ishmael be banished. According to the Koran, Ishmael went to Mecca and his descendants, growing up in Arabia, became Muslims whereas the descendants of Isaac, who stayed in Palestine, became the Jews. According to the orthodox Muslims, Mohammed, the Prophet through whom Islam came into being, was the last, the "Seal of the Prophets", as there will be no more after him. Mohammed was born into the leading tribe of Mecca, the *Koerish*, circa 571 A.D. His life was most difficult. His father died a few days before he was born and his mother also died by the time he became six years old. Thus he was taken into his grandfather's home, who cared for him until he was nine, and finally he went unto his uncle's home where he tended his flock. Poverty forced the young orphan to work hard for a living but the angels apparently opened Mohammed's heart and filled it with Light.

Pure-hearted and well liked, Mohammed had a sweet and gentle disposition. His bereavement and poverty made him sensitive to human suffering of all kinds and he was said to be always ready to help others, the poor and the weak in particular. At that time, conditions in Arabia were very harsh, "barbaric" as they have been described where "might and hedonism were really king"! Upon reaching maturity, Mohammed took up the caravan business and at the age of 25 he entered into the service of a wealthy widow, Khadija whom he later married, even though she was 15 years his senior. She remained true to him to the very end and became one of his first disciples.

Tradition stated that "God comforted him through her and made his burden light". Mohammed soon felt the need for solitude and spent many hours in a cavern on Mount Hira on the outskirts of Mecca. There he meditated on the mysteries of good and evil, unable to accept the sufferings and evil he saw all around him. Through his fasting and vigils, he became convinced that Allah was far greater than his countrymen had supposed and was, literally, the One God, the *True God* without rivals. From this mountain cave, he uttered the cry that was to become the foundation of Islam and to circulate throughout the world, *La ilaha illa Allah!* There is no God but Allah!

As Mohammed's visit to the cave became more frequent, together with his prayers and devotions, he finally received his "commission" from God. As Prof. Smith incisively put it, "It was the same command that had fallen earlier on Abraham, Moses, Samuel, and Jesus. Wherever, whenever this call comes its form may differ but its essence is the same. A voice falls from heaven saying, 'Thou art the man'. On the Night of Power and Excellence, as a strange peace pervaded creation and all nature was turned towards its Lord, in the middle of that night, say the Muslims, the Book was open to a ready soul. As he lay on the floor of the cave, his mind locked in deepest contemplation, a voice commanded Mohammed to cry."

Twice the voice commanded and Mohammed resisted, wishing nothing so much as to escape from the overwhelming Presence. "Cry" commanded the voice for the third time . . . Arousing from his trance, Mohammed felt as if the words he had heard had been branded on his soul. Terrified, he rushed home and fell into paroxysms. Coming to himself, he told Khadija that he had become either a prophet or one possessed—mad . . . "Rejoice, O dear husband, and be of good cheer", she said, "Thou wilt be the Prophet of this people".

From that time onwards, Mohammed's life was no longer his own, it was given to God and to man to preach and bring forth the revelations he had received in spite of relentless persecution, insult, and outrage, and it lasted another 23 years. In a very revealing passage, Huston Smith tells us: "In an age charged with supernaturalism, when miracles were accepted as the stock-in-trade of the most ordinary saint, Mohammed refused to traffic with human weakness and credulity. To miracle-hungry idolaters seeking signs and portents, he cut the issue clean: 'God has not sent me to work wonders. He has sent me to preach to you . . . I am only a preacher of God's words, the bringer of God's message to mankind". If signs be sought, let them not be of Mohammed's greatness but of God's and for these one need only open one's eyes"'.

Mohammed taught that the universe and life were *orderly* and governed by universal and *immutable laws* which led to awaken the Muslim interest and interest in Science long before the Christian West did so. The only true miracle that Mohammed acknowledged was that of the Koran. The response to his message and revelation was, predictably, hostile and this for three basic reasons: his uncompromising monotheism which threatened the Bedouin clergy's revenues from different shrines, his strict moral teachings which denounced the licentiousness of the people, and his democratic social ethic which run counter the unjust and hierarchical economic and social order. The new Prophet's vision that, in the sight of the Lord, all men and women are *equal* really clashed with the well-entrenched nepotism, feudalism, and class-distinctions.

As Prof. Smith described it: "As such teaching suited neither their taste nor their privileges, the Meccan leaders were determined to have none of it. They began their attack with ridicule: laughter, petty insults, and hoot of derision. When these proved ineffective their words took a fiercer turn in abuse, calumny, vilification, and threat. When, these, too, failed, they turned from taunts to open persecution. They covered Mohammed and his followers with dirt and filth while they were engaged in their devotion. They pelted them with stones, beat them with sticks, threw them into prison, and tried to starve them by refusing to sell to them . . . At the sacrifice of all their worldly interests and hopes, and at repeated risks of death itself, followers adhered to the new prophet with a loyalty and devotion seldom paralleled in the world's history."

What began as a visionary claim on the part of a poor and exalted camel-driver later turned into a very serious revolutionary movement that threatened the very foundation of Arab society. Hence the powers that be were determined to silence the troublemaker forever. As he faced his most severe social and personal crisis of his life, Mohammed was visited by a delegation of 75 members of the leading citizens of Yathrib (the modern Medina). As that city was facing severe internal strife and was in need of a strong leader, they turned to Mohammed. After much thought and prevarication, Mohammed told them that he would come on the condition that they worship none but God, observe the precepts of Islam, obey him in all that was right, and defend him as they would their own family. They agreed and Mohammed left for Medina with about 100 of his followers. As he left the City of Mecca being sought by their soldiers, he hid in a ravine with a companion who, in despair, told him something like "we shall never make it as we are only two". Mohammed answered, "No, we are three for God is with us". Three days later, after the search was over, they managed to find camels and leave.

It was the year 622 A.C. and became known in Arabic as the *Hegira* or Great Flight. There Mohammed assumed a different role. From prophet, he now becomes politician and statesman, as the "king" not only of the hearts of a few devotees but of the collective life of a great city, its teacher, governor, judge, and general. Faced with problems of extraordinary complexity, he played his role brilliantly and achieved remarkable success. As Prof. Smith commented: "Supreme magistrate, he continued to lead as he had in the days of his obscurity, an *unpretentious life*. Scorning palaces, he continues to live in an ordinary clay house, milks his own goats, and is accessible day or night to the humblest of his subjects. Often seen mending his own clothes, "no emperor with his tiaras was obeyed as this man in a cloak of his own clouting. God, say the Muslim historians had indeed put before him the key to the treasurers of this world but he refused it." Tradition described his administration as a perfect blend of *justice* (law) with *mercy* (compassion). For the last ten years of life, Mohammed blended his personal biography with the history of Medina. Two Jewish tribes also lived in Medina and enjoyed freedom and social justice.

Many battles were fought between the larger Meccan army and the smaller but more motivated Medinan army. Eighty years after his departure, Mohammed returned to Mecca an undisputed conqueror. Making his way to the Kaaba stone, the center of the religious focus of Mecca, he *forgave his former enemies*, rededicated the stone to Allah, and accepted the mass conversion of the city but then returned to Medina. Two years later, in 632 A.D. he died with practically all of Arabia under his control. As Prof. Smith concluded: "With all the power of armies, police, and civil service, no other Arab had ever succeeded in uniting his countrymen as he had. By the time a century had passed, his followers had conquered Armenia, Persia, Syria, Palestine, Iraq, Egypt, and Spain, and had crossed the Pyrenees into France. But for their defeat by Charles Martel in the Battle of Tours in 732 A.D., the entire Western world might today be Muslim . . . Muslims have a simple explanation. "The entire work", they say, "was the work of God"".

The only miracle that God performed for him, Mohammed claimed, the "standing Miracle", is the Koran which means "to read" or "to recite". Together with the Bible, it is the most read book in the world and certainly the one that is most often committed to memory. It is about 4/5 of the length of the Bible and is divided into 114 chapters or *Surahs*. As far as orthodox Muslim are concerned, every letter of the Koran was directly dictated by God through the single voice that Mohammed heard and which became identified with the Archangel Gabriel. Islam postulates that the Bible of the Jews, the Old Testament, and the Bible of the Christians, the New Testament, are all authentic revelations from God, but which are given different interpretations. This is the reason why Jews, Christians, and Muslims are known as the "People of the Book". Having been revealed at a later time, when humanity was more evolved, functioning at a higher level of consciousness, and untarnished by transmission, the Koran is seen as the definitive Revelation.

As Prof. Smith commented: "The only miracle Mohammed claimed was that he, unschooled to the extent that he could not write his own name, should have produced a book embodying all wisdom and theology essential to human life which in addition is grammatically perfect and without poetic equal". The Koran, written in Arabic, is also one of the most inaccessible religious books to Western religious and philosophical sensibility. According to the orthodox Muslim, it simply cannot be translated and must be read and chanted in Arabic. As an old and famous proverb claims, "Wisdom has alighted on three things: the brain of the Franks, the hands of the Chinese, and the tongue of the Arabs."

The essential theology of Islam is very similar to that of its neighbors, the Jews and Christians. We will look at the four most important ones and their distinctive features for Islam: Allah, Creation, Man, and the Day of Judgment. As with the other high religions, Islam centers on the primal fact of God. Allah is immaterial and thus invisible. The Arabs were already familiar with the invisible world of the spirit. The innovation of the Koran was to focus upon the divine in a single God, a Unified Personal Will, Who overshadows the whole of creation with His Presence and Power. The Jews already had this conception in their famous *Shema*, "Hear O Israel, the Lord our God, the Lord is One" but, for the Muslim, they had reverted to the worship of household gods and golden calves. Christians, on the other hand, have compromised their strict monotheism by deifying Christ. Islam honors Jesus as a true prophet and even accepted His Virgin Birth but rejected the doctrine of the Incarnation and of the Trinity and claim that it is not right for God to have children.

When Jesus claimed to be the Son of God, He was thinking of the Fatherhood of God applying to all of humanity. Every human being, thus you and I, are children of God (at least potentially until spiritual faculties and potentialities are actualized and brought into consciousness). The Koran proclaims, loud and clear, There is no God but He—the Living, the Eternal, the Compassionate one, Allah. As Prof. Smith summarized it: "Allah, then, is one immaterial, all-powerful, all pervading and benevolent. He is also Creator, which brings us to the second basic concept of Islam. In the Islamic conception the world did not emerge, as the Hindus would have it, by some process of emanation from the divine. It was created by a deliberate act of God's Will (He has created the heavens and the earth) . . . . Being the handiwork of a God who is both great and good, the world of matter must, likewise, be basically good".

God's supreme achievement is the *creation of Man*, who is made in His image. It is here that we find the appreciation and value of the individual. As Huston Smith summarized it: "For Islam individuality is not only fully real but also good in principle. As expressed in the human soul it is also eternal, for once created the soul lives forever. Value, virtue, goodness, and spiritual fulfillment come by expressing one's unique self by virtue of which one is different from anyone or anything else. As a great Muslim philosopher has written, "this inexplicable, finite centre of experience is the fundamental fact of the universe. All life is *individual*; there is no such thing as universal life. God Himself is an individual: He is the most unique individual". Islam completely believes in man's freedom and responsibility. Life on earth is but the foundation or "school" for the afterlife, the eternal life. Islam counsels man to walk in the straight path, the path of righteousness.

As Prof. Smith explains, "The straight path is neither crooked not corrupt . . . it is straightforward, direct, and explicit . . . It pinpoints it, nailing it down through explicit injunctions . . . A Muslim knows where he stands. He knows who he is and Who God is. He knows what his obligations are and if he transgresses these he knows what to do about it . . . Islam has a *clarity*, an *order*, a *precision* which is in sharp contrast to the shifting, relative, uncertain, at-sea quality of much of modern life. Muslims explicitly claim this as one of Islam's strengths." Love is the essential key here and thus the question is *how shall we love God and our neighbor?* One last Prophet was required to answer that question who was Mohammed. It is because God Himself answers that question through him that he deserves the title of "the Seal of the Prophets". As a Muslim writer puts it, "the glory of Islam consists in having embodied the beautiful sentiment of Jesus into definite laws"!

In Islam, every person will undergo a final Judgment which will determine whether the soul will go to Heaven or to Hell depending on how it has lived on earth. As the Koran states, "When the sun shall be folded up and the stars shall fall . . . then shall every soul know what it has done . . . Every man's actions have we hung round his neck, and on the last day shall be laid before him a wide-open book". As in other religions, depending on their level of consciousness, this can be taken literally or figuratively with the need for multiple possible explanations. Essentially, the Muslim's view is that each soul will be held accountable for what it has done and how it has lived on earth and whether it has observed God's laws or not.

Theologically and doctrinally, the first pillar of Islam is the creed, "There is no God but Allah, and Mohammed is His Prophet", hence radical monotheism and the assertion that Mohammed was an authentic prophet just as the Koran is a sacred Scripture inspired by God. As Mohammed's successor succinctly put it: "If there are any among you who worship Mohammed, he is dead. But if it is God you worship, he lives forever". The second pillar is *prayer* in which the Koran reminds the faithful to be "constant", that is to pray five times a day. There are many reasons for this but as Prof. Smith explains: "Man is creature rather than creator, man has nevertheless an inveterate tendency to place himself at the center of his universe and live as a law unto himself. When he does so, however, when he tries to play God, everything goes wrong. Man is a creature; his life slips into place in proper perspective only when he recognizes this fact." Muslim can pray *anywhere* but always facing Mecca. The Muslim also washes himself, spreads his pray rug before him and recites the *Sudra* of the Koran, *Allahu Akbar,* God is Great. Finally, the content of Muslim prayer is twofold, the expression of gratitude and praise".

The third pillar of Islam is *charity*. Material things are important in life and some people have more than they need while others less. Those that have more have a moral obligation to help those that have less. In essence, it is the Western modern concept of the *welfare state*. The fourth pillar is the observance of *Ramadan,* fasting during the holy month of Islam in daytime. The fifth and final pillar is a *pilgrimage* to Mecca. As Prof. Smith elucidates, "Once during his lifetime every Muslim who is physically and economically in a position to do so is expected to journey to Mecca where God's climatic revelation was first disclosed. The basic purpose of the pilgrimage is to heighten the pilgrim's devotion to God and to His revealed Will." From my standpoint, it is also a way to heighten a person's consciousness so that some of Mohammed's revelation can also be re-enacted in the pilgrim! It is also useful in international relations and to have a major break in one's daily and secular life.

A final very important concept of Islam is its concept of "Brotherhood". Every Muslim is brother or sister to every other Muslim and should act accordingly. Shortly before his death, Mohammed made a "farewell pilgrimage" Mecca and stated the following which epitomized one of Islam's loftiest ideals and greatest concerns: "O ye men! Harken unto my words and take ye them to heart! Know that every Muslim is a brother to every other Muslim and that you are now one brotherhood!" So the core of Islam is precisely what Jesus and the other genuine prophets always taught, *brotherly love!* Finally, as Huston Smith explains: "Westerners who define religion in terms of *personal experience* would never be understood by Muslims whose religion calls then to establish a very explicit kind of *social order*. Faith and politics, religion and society are inseparable in Islam".

Muslim law covers four basic areas of man's collective life. The first is economic regulation. Islam puts a great deal of emphasis on the physical basis of man's life. In order to be healthy one needs to meet one's physical needs, eating, drinking, housing, and clothing in particular. A major concern of Mohammed was thus to break the barriers of economic caste and to reduce the injustices of special privilege. Competition is necessary but must be balanced by fair play and compassion. Islam also states quite clearly that *unearned money is not one's own.* As Prof. Smith points out: "Every time a Muslim lifts a morsel of food to his mouth he should be able to answer affirmatively the question, 'Have I contributed to the human enterprise sufficiently to deserve what I am now receiving?'".

The second is the status of women. Actually, from existing conditions, Mohammed improved enormously the status of women. He forbade infanticide, he required that daughters be included in inheritance, and opened the way to woman's full equality with men in terms of her rights as citizen: education, suffrage, and vocation. This is not necessarily what Muslim countries and societies practice, but it is *the ideal* towards which they should be aiming. Islam also made marriage the sole condition of the sexual act. While polygamy is still being practiced . . . as it was once practiced all over the world and is now still being practiced by the wealthy, the Koranic law pressures man towards monogamy. As Prof. Smith explains: "There are circumstances in this imperfect state of human existence where polygyny is morally preferable to its alternative. Individually such a condition might arise, for example, if a partner were early in marriage to contract paralysis or another disability which would debar her from sexual union. Collectively, a war which reduced the number of men to half the number of women would be another example."

The third area is *race relations*. Islam emphasizes absolute racial equality showing by their acceptance of racially mixed marriage. Mohammed's second wife, Hagar, was reputed to be black. The fourth and final area is *the use of force.* The Koran does not counsel turning the other cheek or pacifism (but neither do most other religions and states!). It does teach forgiveness and returning good for evil when the circumstances warrant it. The Koran, however, allows punishment to the full extent of the injury and the use of military force to defend one's country and one's self. The Muslims have an interesting concept, that of the *jihad* or holy war. This can be interpreted either in outer or in inner terms, depending on one's level of consciousness and being. In inner, psychological terms, it implies the inevitable conflict or struggle between the higher and the lower self of a person, thus this war is *spiritual in nature.* In outer terms, it means to wage war in the world against infidels in physical terms which, unfortunately, is what happened many times in human history and the history of Islam.

Mohammed also strongly emphasized the principle of religious freedom and acceptance. Thus he stated: "The Jews who attach themselves to our commonwealth have similar rights which were later also mentioned for Christians (these two being the only non-Muslim religions on the scene); these shall be protected from all insults and vexations; they shall have an equal right with our own people to our assistance and good office: the Jews . . . and all others domiciled in Yathrib, shall . . . practice their religion as freely as Muslims." Even conquered nations were given freedom of worship on the condition that they paid a special tax in lieu of the Poor Tax which all Muslims had to pay and from which they were exempt. Interference with liberty of conscience was thus in direct contradiction with Muslim law. As Huston Smith concluded, "There is the heartening story of how during the long centuries of Europe's Dark Ages Muslim philosophers and scientists kept the lamp of learning bright, ready to rekindle the Western mind when it roused from its long sleep."

There is no question that all religions that are truly authentic and that had a world impact, both in space and time, are inspired by a higher Power that, for the absence of a better word, we can call "God". This Power is both internal and external to the persons who receive it, transmit it and live it. Hence, they are truly fundamental for the human condition and play a crucial role in human experience. They are both spiritually inspired and socioculturally influenced and structured, mixing human and trans-human elements. Eastern religions adapted to the Eastern culture, history, and temperament while Western religions did the same for their Western counterpart.

While truly essential is how these "visions, voices, and revelations" were interpreted and applied in human life. And here there are enormous differences between the Founders and their followers, between the Saints and Sages and the people, normal average persons. These differences can point and lead to the *very best* or the *very worst* in human experience, to authentic *love* or passionate *hatred*, to true service and worship or their very opposite Hence, they contain the *opposites* and can manifest these opposites depending not on the religion or doctrine themselves but rather on how they are *interpreted and applied*, which is always a function of the level of consciousness and being of the person who receives them. As such, religion can provide the greatest stimulus for human growth and spiritual evolution or one of their most important obstacles! Beauty and Truth are truly in the "eyes of the beholder" at least in the human experience such as we know it and live at the present time!

Conclusion and synopsis

In the present work and its first part, The Major World Religions, I have attempted to go to the very heart of what human nature, human knowledge, and human destiny really are, of what human beings need and aspire to give meaning and significance to their lives as well as to find the motivation and the fulfillment to continue living. I have taken a very specific "perspective" or "frame of reference" to answer these truly significant questions—that of religion, rather than that of philosophy, literature, or science. To do so, I have attempted to gain closure and describe what the four Eastern World Religions and the three Western World Religions are all about and how they would go about answering these truly essential questions.

In so doing, I have, obviously, left out more than I have included and I have presented these materials as they were researched by Prof. Huston Smith and interpreted and synthesized from my point of view. All the quotes and basic materials were drawn from his book, *The Religions of Man* (Perennial Library, Harper & Row, 1958) which I highly recommend. Much is, therefore, omitted and not covered but it is my hope that what is truly essential, the substance or *quintessence* of these mainstream traditions have been included and represented in a simple, direct, and impartial way. Bearing in mind what Justice Homes once said, "that Science gives very complete and practical answers to unimportant questions whereas religion gives incomplete and abstract answers to truly fundamental questions"; and that Religion properly understood and applied—that is approached from a higher level of consciousness and being—can indeed provide most important and useful information, I have embarked on this fascinating and very illuminating journey of exploring, from a personal and spiritual viewpoint, the contributions of humanity's main religions to the truly fundamental questions of human Life.

This journey and study, which are far from being exhaustive or even objective, should at least provide a good *spring-board* for your own reflection and analysis of what we can gather from Religion concerning human nature, knowledge, and destiny, what human beings need and aspire to and what they strive to realize in their earthly pilgrimage. This endeavor and journey is fraught with paradoxes, contradictions, and difficulties which, however, characterize *la condition humaine*, as the French call it. I have found that there are certain basic insights, intuitions, ideas, and "keys" that can greatly help to make sense of this complex and contradictory material as well as to reconcile and integrates opposites. These are the following which I would invite you all to reflect upon, to master and then apply to your own study and reflection of the truly *fundamental questions of Life:*

1. The analogy and correspondence between the microcosm (Man) and the Macrocosm (the universe). Ancient wisdom and the Hermetic tradition in particular, as well as the realizations and teachings of the great Mystics, have always claimed that a human being is truly a "mirror" or "reflection" of all there is; that there is nothing outside of human nature that is not in human nature and vice versa. Thus, if there are three basic entities and dimensions in the outer world—God, Humanity and Nature, or the physical, psychosocial, and psychospiritual dimensions—these must also be found (and they are) in *human nature*—the Spirit, Pneuma, or spiritual Self, the soul, psyche, or human consciousness, and the biological organism. And, if we wish to become aware of, perceive, interact, and make exchanges with what is *outside of us* we must first *awaken and activate its corresponding part within ourselves!*

    What this means, in a nutshell, is that anything that ever occurred in the *world* and in *history* must also occur within *ourselves in the present.* Hence, what religions are really about is not so much the Prophets, Saints, Sages or Avatars of the past and past cultural and historical events as they are about what we can *awaken, activate and live within ourselves at the psychospiritual level.* This is a truly fundamental "esoteric" or wisdom "key" that can shed a great deal of light upon what is truly important and practical about religion. The aphorism that best represents this insight is the famous saying of Angelus Silesius, "Should Jesus Christ a thousand times in Bethlehem be born but not in my soul, I would still be lost"! It is this insight and realization that best characterizes and separates the *exoteric* or outer aspect of religion and its *esoteric* or inner aspect that constitutes the heart of the "religion of the Saints and Sages".

2. The ultimate "key" to understand human nature, the universe, Life, God, or anything lies within human nature itself and the psyche is *human consciousness!* Without a proper understanding of human consciousness, its nature, dynamics, and manifestations all the rest remains fatally vitiated and distorted. There is a way, an "essential gate" through which the growth and development of all knowledge,

understanding, and wisdom must go through to answer the truly "fundamental questions" of Life and that is *the transformation and expansion of human consciousness*! Just like the universe is expanding with galaxies and star systems moving away from each other, so human consciousness is also growing and expanding, not only at the horizontal (quantitative) but also at the vertical (qualitative) level and it is here that we will find the answers to our questions or fail to find them! Every problem, every question does have an answer but this answer may lie on a higher level (of consciousness) than the one in which the problem of question was formulated.

3. The human sky-scraper and the vertical axis of consciousness. This is another truly fundamental insight and "explanatory key" to properly understand not only religion but many of the paradoxes and contradictions of the human condition. I have received and elaborated this insight for several years, embodying it in a book in two volumes, entitled, "L'Homme Gratte-Ciel", (Les Editions de l'Aigle, 2000)—*Man, the Sky-Scraper*. The core assumption here is that *Reality and Truth are really functions of our level of consciousness and being, of our evolution*! As there are seven possible levels of consciousness and being with four being the more diffused and "practical ones", there really are seven very different ways of *perceiving, conceiving and reacting to the very same thing!*

If we take the human life-cycle as our point of reference, there are babies, infants, adolescents, young adults, adults, mature adults, and older persons who perceive, conceive, and react to the same things in a very different way! Moreover, each human being must go through and live the entire range! There is no way that a baby can become an adolescent without first being and living as a child or that an adolescent can become a mature adult without first being and living as an adult!

Properly understood this core idea will show us why it is so important to *forgive others and ourselves,* to aspire and strive for perfection but without expecting to achieve it, and to be tolerant and compassionate for others who are still prey to weaknesses and defects that may not affect us! Human beings are still *imperfect beings living in an imperfect world* and, as such, they must all learn how to cope with fear, anxiety, and guilt, with the limitations of the ego as well as with sexual and aggressive energies, frustrations and rage. These are part and parcel of our human experience, at this point in our evolution, but can eventually be transcended.

4. There are very important semantical differences between the language of everyday speech, the language of science, and the language of religion and poetry! While the terms may be the same, be written and pronounced

in the same way, the meanings, implications and applications attached to them are very different.

The language of everyday speech utilizes *words* which are instruments or media designed to convey and elicit thoughts (denotations) and emotions (connotations). The language of science utilizes *concepts* which are instruments or media designed to convey and elicit only thoughts (ideally one denotation with an empirical deferens). The language of religion and poetry utilizes *symbols* which are instruments or media designed to convey and elicit thoughts, feelings and intuitions. Thus symbols can have as many different meanings, implications and applications, as there are different levels of consciousness and symbols, words, and concepts should never be confused or seen as being identical.

5. There is a fundamental difference between *knowledge* and *understanding* that is what we have learned through our own direct personal experience and what we have read or thought out mentally. The more profound religious insights and ideas and all spiritual truths must be *lived* and not only *thought out* to be properly understood. This is what distinguishes the Eastern Orthodox Church and the Roman Catholic Church in the Christian tradition. The first took Plato is its basic "frame of reference and Model" whereas the second aligned itself with Aristotle, thus emphasizing *direct, lived experience*, which one must prepare for and be guided towards by spiritual elders, or *rational, scholarly knowledge* which can be gotten out of seminaries and universities!

6. The founders and leaders of all authentic world religions and traditions were *exceptional people with exceptional gifts and faculties* which, ultimately, can only be properly understood and appreciated by those who have developed the same. Hence, their *vision*, conception and interpretation, as well as the incarnation or living of their visions, revelations, and intuitions are quite different than those of their followers which, sometimes, may also be opposite. Example, they first are almost always non-violent, humble, and quite compassionate towards others where as the second can often be violent, arrogant, and cruel!

Bearing in mind the image and analogy of the human sky-scraper, however, we can easily understand how people on different level of consciousness and evolution can perceive and define the same thing in very different ways. Not only, but that each and every human being must go through all phases of human evolution. Hence, we must all be "babies", "infants", and "adolescents" before we can become "adults" or "older persons". Thus the need for tolerance, flexibility, humility, and forgiveness—for looking at things from the standpoint of *eternity* rather than in temporal terms!

7. Learn to properly understand, integrate, and *live* the two essential "axes" of authentic spirituality—*Prayer* (the love of God) and *Service* (the love of our fellow humans beings).

8. Learn how to properly understand and integrate the *masculine and feminine polarities*, spirit and matter, the outer and the inner, in our consciousness and in our lives.

9. Learn to give priority to *Love* rather than to Knowledge or Power so as to be able to move from knowledge to wisdom and to integrate the two.

10. Properly understand and apply the "parable of the Prodigal Son" to ourselves and our present historical period. We are all the "Prodigal Son", the "solar hero"! We left our true home, the "spiritual worlds", to slowly move down the planes of creation to incarnate in the physical world. Now, however, we have to begin our return journey to those "spiritual worlds" and our true Self.

    Now (at the end of the 20th and the beginning of the 21st centuries) we are truly "hitting bottom"; that is we could not descend lower into the physical, material world and into the restricted world of our human self—into *egoism*. Thus, a truly major transition and transformation is, indeed, upon us, with a radical change of orientation, values, and priorities. The slow process of "secularization" and of "analyzing smaller and smaller units" must now be replaced and integrated with the process of "spiritualization" and of "synthesis": uniting disparate parts into larger and larger whole.

11. We must also begin to realize that the true "secret" of Self and Life—and of all the questions that are truly important—can never be found in *Matter* and its analysis but only in *Life* and *Consciousness* and their proper integration and understanding!

12. Last but not least, we have the image and analogy of the "House of Science" which can be very useful and shed a great deal of light in properly understanding where we are, where we are coming from, and where we are going in terms of *valid knowledge*. We now stand at a very crucial "turning point" where a new group of sciences—*Spiritual Science*—is in the process of emerging and being born. It is only when this new group of sciences will be fully articulated that we will obtain the full and holistic picture of what we are, where we are coming from, and where we are going; why the spiritual dimension slowly "faded away" from our conscious awareness and preoccupation only to be "reborn" and "reintegrated" at a later time.

Human beings truly are very complex, incomplete and paradoxical beings who want very different things—even opposed things—at different levels of consciousness, being, and evolution. First, they want to su*rvive*, biologically, psychologically, socially but then also spiritually. Then, they want to *realize their goals and ideals* which vary accordingly . . . First, they want to satisfy the basic needs and aspirations or desires of their egos: essentially, health, wealth, love and worldly success. Then, however, when they realize that the above will never bring full and lasting satisfaction, they want to understand and do God's Will—the will of their spiritual Self. Rather than working for the "part", eventually, they want to work for the "whole" even if this requires effort and sacrifices, "long-term goals" rather than "short-term goals"!

What human beings really want is *Life, Love,* and *Knowledge;* being able to answer the "Riddle of the Sphinx", know who they are and why they came in this world—what is really important to accomplish in this life. They want to know God's Will, the will of their own higher Self, and what is their destiny, why they have incarnated in this world. They also want to be able to love and be loved, to feel deeply and passionately, to be inspired and come alive by connecting and uniting with something that is greater than they are! And they want to be able to express themselves, to create, to make a difference in this world!

Religion (the means) and spirituality (the end) can be extremely important and make truly essential contributions to what human beings need and want the most so, when they are *authentic*, they carry forth and transmit an inestimable *treasure* but a treasure which must be properly understood, integrated in one's life and personality, and *lived* rather than being merely "known" or "reflected upon". There are many religions because these are the different paths that lead to the same goal or "summit" and which reflect the different levels of consciousness and being, culture, personality, and history of different people. But there is *one authentic spirituality* with many levels and facets just like a diamond is one stone but with many facets! Today, religion, whichever it might be, faces a very important problem and dilemma which will determine whether it will wane away and become irrelevant or go through a major spiritual Renaissance: it must relate the letter with the spirit, the exoteric with the esoteric aspects, the religion of the people with that of the Saints and Sages, for this is what our present level of consciousness and evolution demand!

I want to make a clear two very important points at the conclusion of the first part of this work that deals with a very brief and pointed representation of the world's major religions. First, it is essential to be able to distinguish between the academic and cognitive study of religion and joining and living a given religion. I do not recommend *syncretism* or making a "cocktail" of various religions, not even seeking the nectar or very best from different religions, for that only leads to confusion and dispersion. As religion deals primarily with love, it is very important to make a choice, then a commitment, and finally to live that love and religion.

The analogy is like looking for a mate: there are many beautiful and worthy men and women in the world. When one is ready, one has to find *one person*, become committed to that person and then live with that one special person. The same is true for religion! This, I believe, has been one of the most important pitfalls of the so-called New Age and of various esoteric or spiritual schools: to seek to blend in and draw upon many different traditions. While it is important to have an *intellectual understanding* of the many religions it is even more important to *incarnate and live* one of them!

Second, I do not advocate or seek to convert anyone to anything and least of all to my or any other religion. Eastern religions and traditions have generally understood and practiced this showing great tolerance and respect for different religions as did the Roman Empire at its height. Western religions, Christianity and Islam in particular, have not understood this and have embarked on the conversion, many times by force, of large numbers of people showing incredible ethnocentrism, intolerance, and arrogance leading to religious wars or conquests with catastrophic results. If a person is born into a given religion, and most people are, my clear and explicit aim is to help them *know and live their tradition* in its deeper levels, implications and applications.

I do not believe that people are born into a given race, culture or religion by "chance" hence they need to bring to fruition that which their soul has chosen! After all, there is one God, one Spiritual Family, and one Wisdom Tradition but which has many facets and manifestations depending on the level of consciousness and being and on the culture and evolutionary level of different people. Tolerance, self-respect, and true charity are thus to be extended to all especially in our day and age when we are, finally, moving from a tribal to a universal religion.

The only true "conversion" or *metanoia* is an *inner and personal one* that must be reached and lived in one's *heart and consciousness*! This occurs many times and in different ways as people move from one level of consciousness to another, from one "floor" of the "inner sky-scraper" to a higher one. The best modern example of this is that of Gladys Hayworth who, though a Christian missionary in China, never sought to convert anyone but ended up by converting the notables of the town where she lived by the kind of courage, integrity, and love that she displayed over many years and facing many extraordinary trials and difficulties. Thus, as there is an "exoteric" form of religion and an "esoteric" one so there is also an "exoteric" and "esoteric" form of conversion!

The true answer to the "religious problem", at least for me, is to remain true to one's religion while, at the same time, respecting and learning from the religions of others—not an easy thing to accomplish! Realizing, however, that there different levels of consciousness and evolution, it should be easy to understand that there is also a need for different religions and denominations, each with its own emphasis and focus. There is also another very interesting side to religion which is that of *revealed* and that of *natural* religion.

Natural religion is the product of the insights and of the genius of a given person whereas revealed religion is the manifestation in human consciousness of a higher Reality and Truth. Another way of putting this is to ask: "does God make man in His own image or does man make god in his image?" I believe that both are true! Up to the *personality level* (until the level of what I call the "man of Talent" or the adolescent) religion can only be *natural* and it is man who makes god in his own image. It is only when the *soul level* is reached (passing what I call the "disciple" level to that of the "Sage") that religion is truly *revealed* when we realize that it is God that makes man in His own image. This is another way of saying that the level of consciousness and being of a person is truly crucial in terms of how they conceive or create and live their religion!

Religions, being based on the double axis of the love of God (Prayer and Worship) and the love of our fellow humans (Service) can focus upon and give primacy to the *inner*, psychological and spiritual life, or to the *outer* life in the world, to spiritual exercises, prayer and rituals, or to social action and the quest for human rights and justice. One is the life of the Monk and Hermit, the other that of the moral and social Reformer. One wishes to prepare the way to enter the "Kingdom of God" which is not of this world while the other seeks to transform this world into "God's Kingdom". For the first a life of purification and consecration, and the practice of psychospiritual exercises, is fundamental, the spiritual experience being an inner *personal* one. For the second, on the other hand, ethics, politics, and human rights are fundamental.

For the first religion deals fundamentally with the inner life and should be kept divorced from the politics and from the state. For the second religion deals with the outer and collective life where the state and politics are an essential part of religion and cannot be divorced from it. Of course both polarities are important and must, somehow, be integrated with each other. Jung would say that the "introvert" would focus upon the inner life and devotion while the "extravert" would privilege the outer life and social action. Personally, I feel that the inner life has primacy and should be our starting point in that what we do in the world is always a projection of what takes place within ourselves and in our consciousness.

Then there is the question of how to interpret and apply the basic symbols, parables, and teachings of a given religion: in a *literal way* or in a *symbolic analogical way*? The fundamentalist or integralist would answer in a literal way while the philosopher and the mystic would, generally, answer in a symbolic and analogical way. For the first, things are relatively simple, there is one right interpretation which was directly inspired by God and which must be adhered to. For the second, things are far more complex in that each person, at each basic level of consciousness and being, must interpret and apply these symbols and teachings in a *personal* way.

The first demands *conformity* and *obedience* and its main problem is religious compliance whereas the second demands a great deal of *work and of personal interpretation and application* and, in particular, to listen to one's own heart, to be true to one's self, and to develop character and integrity. I also see this dichotomy in terms of the level of consciousness and being of the person. The child must learn and obey while the adult must make up his own mind and then assume responsibility for his positions actions.

Henri Bergson, the Nobel Laureate in Philosophy/Literature, developed a very interesting conception and distinction between *static* and *dynamic* religion and morality. Static religion and morality are primarily concerned with *avoiding doing evil* even at the cost of not experimenting or doing much. Dynamic religion and morality, on the other hand, are primarily concerned with *doing good*, with experimenting even at the cost of making mistakes and of doing evil. As we are incomplete beings living in an incomplete world, where the most important thing is to grow, mature and make progress, I feel that static religion and morality are far less evolved and progressive than dynamic religion and morality which is why Bergson states that the first was the position of the people and the second, the position of the mystics. The first would apply a strict justice with little compassion or forgiveness while the second would strongly emphasize compassion and the ability to forgive, both others and oneself!

According to the spiritual tradition, the greatest and most sacred attribute of a human being in this world is *free will*—the ability to choose. This means many things one of which is certainly that one is *free to choose between good and evil* and that one can *learn from both!* Doing evil in this world of duality brings death, suffering, unconsciousness, and slavery whereas going good brings life, joy, consciousness and freedom. Our human potential and the range of our possible experimentation and actions is far greater than anything that our best minds can possibly imagine at this point thus we will try out, carry out, and do all kinds of things both great and terrible, human and inhuman, good and evil. But, there is a fundamental principle that claims that whatsoever we do unto others always comes back so that, in the end, we do it *unto ourselves*! Hence, if we don't want something to happen to ourselves, we should not do it to others!

Another truly essential point is whether a human being is basically a *mortal, physical, being* or an *immortal, spiritual being?* Whether all there is to human existence and life is carried out in this world between birth and death or whether there is a much greater existence and life that human beings can access in the spiritual worlds? Whether we are *alone* in the universe or whether there are an infinity of beings who are more or less evolved than we are with One Creator and Father of all? Most religions, most of the time, with the exception of the modern psychological or political religions (psychoanalysis and communism), have argued for a *trans-empirical frame of reference*. They have claimed and taught that the spiritual is causal and primary to the physical, that religion is far more metaphysical than ethical in its nature, and that we are not alone in the universe!

One thing, however, is sure: should a human being be a mortal being where all there is to his life and existence is what transpires between birth and death in this world, then the human condition and experiment would be the most abject failure and tragedy as most people, most of the times, have very difficult and "unjust lives" where they can neither "know themselves" or truly "express themselves". On the other hand, should a human being be an immortal being and life in this world be a "school" or "laboratory" for his becoming and self-actualization, then *all human situations*, even the most painful and "unjust" become transformed and redeemed, assuming true meaning, purpose, and value.

La *bêtise humaine* (human foolishness), which has been said to be infinite and without remedy, can then be seen in a very different and more tolerant light: "They don't know what they are doing; they are playing dangerous games, but they will learn from all their mistakes" . . . My position is that a human being is and has always been *an immortal, spiritual being* but that he has lost the consciousness of his immortality which is what he must and will reacquire!

There is one final and most important point, I would like to mention before closing this most interesting exploration and study of religions and their contributions to human well-being and evolution. There is one thing that is truly very simple and essential and that is that human beings have incarnated in this world to learn, to grow, to mature—*to make progress* or become more than what they were when they were born! And there is no doubt that everyone, in spite of one's personal situation, position, choices, and type as well as length of life, will learn, grow, mature and make progress through what they have experienced in the physical world!

Joy and sorrow, pleasure and pain, peace and anxiety, love and hatred, are all powerful existential "motivators" for our own growth and progress. The most important thing is not so much *what happens to us* as how *we perceive, define, and react to what happens to us!* The important thing is to learn how to live with peace, gratitude, and joy for the extraordinary gift we have been given in this world to *become more than what we are;* and to realize that, in the end, when we have achieved higher states of consciousness and become who we truly are, we will be able to say: *it has been WORTH-WHILE* . . . as it was necessary for me to go through "all of this" in order to become what I now AM! This, at least, is the living testimony of the founders of all great world religions as well as the teaching of all the authentic Mystics, Saints and Sages . . . that **you** will also be able to verify and experience when you reach their level of being and evolution . . . which is your destiny!

PART II

Religion and Spirituality,
their relationship and distinctive
characteristics

Introduction

In the first part of this work, we have claimed that we live in a very special, "abnormal" historical period characterized by massive quantitative and qualitative change and transformation. Essentially what characterizes this historical juncture, from the standpoint of the spiritual perspective, is the fact that we are no longer children while not being adults yet. Thus we are living through our "crisis of adolescence" where we experiment wildly with everything, wanting to test and benefit from the newly discovered powers of our minds and wills! The Fall (or involution of the spirit into matter) and its impact on our consciousness and memory has brought us to conclude that we are alone in the universe, that our existence and becoming are the product of random chance and evolution, and that everything depends on us, on what we can or cannot do for ourselves with our intelligence and human resources. It has led to a much narrowed view of Life and reality as being essentially *material* in nature and thus where egoism, selfishness, and egocentrism are the iron law of reality.

We have witnessed and described the incredible paradox and contradiction that human beings have never had *so much* (education, knowledge, technology, money, and consumer goods) and yet they have never been so *confused, miserable, and depressed* (as measured by the statistics of suicide, psychopathology, anti-social behavior, and depression to mention only the most important ones)! This, I suggested, was to the fact that modern man has "conquered the world (projected himself into the outer, physical world to harness its energies and materials to satisfy the needs and desires of his ego) but lost his own soul (the deeper sense of meaning, purpose, and value of himself, of his life, and opportunities in the physical world)". Many great world leaders and thinkers have given us a very clear and serious warning in the second half of the 20th century, to cite just a few:

- "Modern civilization has built huge sky-scrapers and powerful machines, but what has it done for the men and women who live in these buildings and who use these machines?" Walt Whitman

- "Life and Evolution are now giving us a very simple and basic choice: rise to a higher level of consciousness and being or destroy yourselves at your own hands". Pitirim Sorokin
- "Modern civilization is headed for *der Enstzaberung der Welt* (for the disenchantment with the world)". This means that with the development of reason and science we will get, in the end, everything that we want, but that nothing will have meaning, purpose and bring true fulfillment. Max Weber
- "The 21st Century will either be spiritual . . . or will not be". André Malraux
- "What shall it profit a man if he gains the whole world but loses his own soul" Jesus of Nazareth (Who said this already 2,000 years ago!).

In a nutshell, we saw and discussed the fact that as human consciousness is expanding and transforming itself, everything that we experience is being intensified, accelerated, and "psychologized" (meaning that it takes place in our own consciousness and is a question of *perception* rather than occurring in the world and being of a material nature); hence that the *very best* and the *very worst*, heaven and hell, as it were, are now manifesting themselves in the world. To make it, survive and thrive, in the 21st century, we will need all of our resources and get all the help we can both at the internal and at the external level. Human suffering as well as human joy and fulfillment are both being amplified and intensified. How to cope with the omni-present human suffering and how to develop the best and highest within ourselves and in our world is thus a truly fundamental issue that needs to be addressed by all who are living today.

Very briefly, I stated how I began to look at the question of human suffering by turning to the economic aspect, then by turning to the political aspect, and finally turning to education and research. In the end, however, I found these lacking and being unable to truly provide an essential solution, important and useful as they are. Thus I turned to *religion*, remembering that one of them, Buddhism, had made the understanding and overcoming of human suffering its essential objective. This led me to come to the conclusion that of all institutions and perspectives, religion was the one that truly held the answer and the effective remedy. But that religion had to be explored not only at the "exoteric" level and in terms of its "letter" but also and especially at the "esoteric" level and in terms of its "spirit". That we had to reunite the "letter" and the "spirit" of religion, its exoteric and esoteric aspects, or the religion of the people with the religion of the Saints and Sages, which may be the same but interpreted and lived in a different fashion.

Thus, I embarked on a brief study and description of the seven major world religions taking the outstanding work of Dr. Huston Smith, *The Religions of Man*, as my main point of reference. This to get at the most essential historical and doctrinal aspects of these religions. Thus I concluded and tried to show why the ultimate answer to all of the fundamental questions of human life, the enigma of the Sphinx and the question of human suffering and destiny in particular, lies in *the transformation and expansion of human consciousness*; this, in turn, required a passage from the outer, horizontal dimension to the inner vertical one and thus reconnecting and reuniting *religion* (which are many and which can only be the means) with *spirituality* (which is one and which is the true end). To do this, we need to look at religion and spirituality, their essential nature, basic characteristics, and relationship. This will be the central focus and goal of the second part of this work.

Basically put, in terms of the level of consciousness and being that most of us have achieved today, religion is the *means* whereas spirituality is the *end*. Thus, you can be religious but not spiritual or spiritual but not overly religious, or you can be both, depending on your level of consciousness and being and thus on the way you look at reality. In this perspective, religion is not essential for salvation (which must be properly understood and realized) but spirituality is. Religion can be taught and transmitted to others while authentic spirituality can only be lived and personally experienced. Finally, religion and spirituality, like any other aspect of Reality, are a trinity with a *body* (a physical or material aspect), a *soul* (human meaning and significance), and a *spirit* (life and power). For religion and spirituality to work and bear fruit, these three aspects must be properly understood and related to each other. While their body and the spirit are still viable and healthy, it is their *soul* that really needs to be worked upon to bring it in line with our present level of consciousness and evolution and to be adapted to and applied by each individual person.

Let us bear in mind one of the great contributions of the sociology of religion; namely, that each religion consists of five *interrelated and interacting systems*: a belief system, a ritual system, and ethical system, an organizational system, and a direct, personal experience system. In most of the Western religions, Catholicism and Protestantism in particular as far as Christianity is concerned, it is the fifth system that has mostly fallen by the wayside, which is lacking, and which must be reinstituted if religion is to survive and go through a major rebirth in the 21st century. This implies an "eldership" or spiritual teacher-student relationship, taking a deep look at one's entire life and how we live it, and a system of *spiritual exercises* to be practiced regularly; what can be found in the monastic experience at its best, but which can also lived and expressed in the world.

In the first chapter of this second part of our work, I will attempt to present you with a specific spiritual interpretation and application of the basic ideas and core insights of Christianity so as to render clear, comprehensible and applicable some of its great treasures, both theoretical and practical. In the second chapter, "the Church, the image of human nature", I will put forth the well-known esoteric insight that one of the most promising and fruitful interpretation of the concept of "Church", or "Temple", is that it represents a *picture*, or blue-print, of *human nature*. The "living Church", in other words, is never a material building or even an association of persons but rather our *own nature*, soul, psyche and body that will then interact and make exchanges with those of other beings. Practically speaking, this means that when a person enters into a Church or a material temple, what he really does is to *enter within his own being and psyche* or consciousness. The external structure, if built according to the principles of sacred geometry and of universal symbolism, really gives us a blue-print of our own anatomy and physiology!

This perspective and view-point clearly opens up a very interesting series of analogies, correspondences, and associations that can be extremely fruitful for practical spiritual work. Most important, it shows quite explicitly that there is a lot of personal work and achievements to be undertaken and that *no one* can do this work, the Great Work, for us. Moreover, it is in complete harmony with the teachings and affirmations of the great Mystics, Saints, and Sages of many religions, traditions, times, and places. One of the best known ones comes from St. Augustine who stated, in his *Confessions*, "Lord, I sought you in all the temples and religions of the world and I did not find you. But, lo and behold, I found you within myself and then I also found you everywhere in the world!" This chapter is thus a very good way to begin applying the insights, concepts, and tools developed in the first chapter.

In the third chapter, "The Christmas Story", I will continue the same work of interpreting and applying our basic insights, assumptions, and tools to a very fundamental insight and archetype of the Christian tradition, that of Christmas. Here, the core insights and fundamental thesis are the same as those of the previous chapter. The real "Christmas", the one that is most important and meaningful for me, is not so much something that happened in the world, in history, and to other people as it is the symbolic and analogical representation of the *birth of spiritual consciousness* within *each one of us*. Thus the real "Christmas" is not so much something that happened in the past and in the world as it is something that must happen to *each one of us* and that will take place in the *future*.

All persons, the events, the images and symbols of this "story" must be translated and applied in terms of the microcosm, of our own self and now! This, obviously, takes time, work, preparation and inspiration, but if we do it correctly and persevere, the rewards and results can truly be extraordinary, way beyond anything that words can really describe. "Christmas" is thus the psychospiritual process by which we become one with Christ and by which spiritual consciousness is born within our own being and consciousness. In symbols and images, it describes the process of our *theosis* or deification, the final stage and greatest objective of the Eastern Orthodox Church. The manger represents our heart center just as Joseph and Mary symbolize the male and female principles, human effort and grace respectively. Once we properly grasp the basic interpretative "key" and the tools to work with, this perspective opens up a fabulous vista and work that we can and must do, when we are ready for it, in order to accomplish the Great Work.

The fourth chapter, "The Story of Easter", the archetype of Resurrection, continues and completes the same psychospiritual process by moving onto and proposing another major celebration and mandala, or set of archetypes of the Christian tradition—that of Easter or of Resurrection. The reader having familiarized himself/herself with our basic perspective and its essential tools, described in the first chapter and illustrated and applied in the second and third ones, should now find it easy to work with them and to apply them to this culminating point of the Christian tradition. In this perspective, Easter is really the symbolic description and celebration (or bringing about) of *rebirth*, at the level of nature and of the personality, and of *resurrection*, at the level of the *soul*. Likewise, it is something that each person must work for, live, and experience for *himself/herself* and not something that occurs in the world, in history, or to someone else—even though the images, the symbols, and the archetypes do come from the outside world.

Each year, therefore, there is something that we can do to facilitate our "rebirth" (a cleansing, tune-up, and revitalization) at the physical, emotional, and mental level of our personality. The effects of this work will last for several months but will then have to be repeated with the coming of each New Year. This will go on until, one day, once we reach our soul level, we will experience an inner "resurrection" at that level, which is indescribable in human words, and which will change and transform us forever, being the true and final culminating point of human evolution and of the earthly experience.

The fifth chapter, "Grace or spiritual energy", will seek to gain closure on a most important kind of energy that science is just now beginning to discover; a spiritual energy that mystics have apprehended as manifesting itself as Light, Fire and Life which is the very ground and matrix or source of all that is: the universe and life. This energy originates at the very core of Reality or God, hence at the divine level, but it can descend through the planes and dimensions of being all the way to the material level, permeating and thus having an impact on the spiritual, the mental, the emotional, the vital, and the physical level. In the Christian tradition, at the higher and more global level, it is known as the "Power of the Holy Spirit"; in other traditions and at a lower and more specific level it is known as "Chi" (China, Japan), "Prana" (India), "Manna" (Polynesia), "vital energy" (the traditional medical system), "Vril", etc.

Here, I will attempt to describe the nature, dynamics, role and contributions of this higher and more subtle form of energy and life and then relate it to human effort in so far as human life and the completion of the Great Work are concerned. Obviously, grace is a free and ineffable gift from God and, ultimately, remains a mystery. There are some aspects, modalities, and manifestations that have occurred historically and that have been described and lived by the Saints, Sages, and Mystics who were its recipients. I have also had some personal experiences of it in my own life and continue doing so on a deepening and intensifying way. Finally, science is now on the threshold of discovering, studying and experimenting with this qualitative form of subtle energy.

The sixth chapter, "Quintessential Christianity", will seek to get to the very heart and core of the Christian tradition, interpreted as a manifestation of the *Hagia Sophia* or Ageless Wisdom, to what is truly essential and what can be distilled and applied in the 21st century to help us meet the enormous challenges to the human spirit that this century will bring to all of us. For we now stand at a truly crucial "cross roads" and major "turning point" of human evolution wherein we must grow and move on, cease being unconscious, mischievous, and destructive children and become conscious, autonomous, and responsible adults. To do this we must pass what I like to call our "adolescence crisis" or "maturity exam" which is what most people will have to face and confront in this century. Here the Holy Wisdom, the spiritual tradition and "quintessential Christianity" have much to contribute.

More and more, I gather evidence and become convinced that without grace, spiritual Light or energy, without higher laws, energies and faculties, than our reason and the five senses of the "black box" of traditional science, we will not be able to meet these challenges and to make it in the 21st century. We are not alone in this universe and neither are our lives and experiences *chaotic* and the product of random chance. It is high time that we realized this that we learn and apply, LIVE, the great laws of Life, God and our own Being . . . if we are to avoid the great dangers and profit from the even greater opportunities that our historical juncture offers us. A proper understanding and use of what *grace* or spiritual Light, and the Ageless Wisdom have to offer are absolutely essential for us to continue our evolutionary journey.

The seventh and final chapter, the "New Encyclopedia: a Compendium of Human Knowledge for the 21st Century", attempts to bring together and to relate to each other, all the knowledge that is available at this historical juncture and that can be gleaned from the spiritual tradition, religion and spirituality. This to offer us a rational and cognitive "road-map" to make sense of all the paradoxes, the contradictions, and the challenges that are thrown at us and which are necessary for us to make sense and be able to integrate the ever-growing range of human experience that we are living through.

Human beings have a definite and essential need to understand and to be able to explain what they experience, to find meaning, purpose and value in what they are living through. If they do, they can make it through the most difficult and painful experiences. If they don't, it is easy for them to "dissociate" and "crack up" psychologically even under relatively normal difficulties or out of boredom. *Logotherapy*, the new school of psychotherapy developed by Viktor Frankel, has very exhaustively and rationally demonstrated this fundamental insight.

This seven and final chapter highlights the essential insights, principles, and assumptions that are necessary to bring about what I have termed the "New Encyclopedia", the synthesis of human knowledge and its interconnections that we need to function properly in the 21st century and to take a our next step in our evolution and self-actualization. It will definitely be a synthesis of religion, science and philosophy which might or might not be perceived as the "religion of the Holy Spirit". Crucial here, will be the ability of religion to relate its exoteric with its esoteric aspects, the "letter" with the "spirit" and the religion of the masses with that of the Saints and Sages.

Science will have to include a spiritual dimension that will complement and complete its physical and psychosocial dimensions and philosophy will again be compelled to direct its attention to the truly crucial questions of humanity and not merely on its inner dynamics or trivial aspects. And of all of this will be made possible when enough men and women raise their level of consciousness to the point where their intuition can be activated and where spiritual consciousness can be awakened, and where they will observe the essential rules of the scientific method which are to focus upon direct *personal observation and experience* and to let the "facts" speak for themselves and be the foundation for theory creation.

Chapter I

RELIGION AND SPIRITUALITY IN THE 21ST CENTURY

Religion and spirituality have always been are still are very closely connected, interconnected, and interacting but, they are not the same thing. Essentially, I believe that religion is the *means*: the instruments and the path which, when properly understood and applied, can lead to the *end* which is spirituality. Religion is the container, the vessel or "temple", the *lamp*, whereas spirituality is the life, the energy, or the "dweller of that temple", the *light*. While it is possible for a person to be religious and not be spiritual and for a person to be spiritual but not religious, obviously the ideal would be to unite the two in an interacting cycle or feedback-loop which is both dynamic and linked with the practitioner's level of consciousness and evolution.

Religion used to be the *via regia* to truth and reality and the most prestigious social institution so long as humanity was still in its "childhood period" and had to be guided and protected by more evolved human beings that acted *in loco parenti* or as their parents and guides. During that long period of time, primitive and traditional (so called) societies where still quite vertical and hierarchical. The chief virtue of the child was obedience, compliance and affection for his parents. During that period of time, the "Great Chain of Being" was still preserved and faith in a higher Power than man was taken for granted. Each person had "his/her place" in the family and in society and the goal was to preserve *justice* or harmony. This implied the *golden mean*: the right measure, the right proportion, the right timing and distance—the right relationship.

Then humanity continued on its evolutionary journey and reached the period of "adolescence" when the basic rules, values and priorities changed dramatically. This occurred rather recently or about 500 years ago (at the time of the Renaissance, followed by the Age of Reason, the Reformation, the French

Revolution, and the Modern Age). Adolescents are notorious for rebelling and rejecting authority, their parents, the experts, and the establishment. They want to become *independent* (while yet remaining dependent), they want to develop their own ways and values and especially they want to *experiment with everything* anew to learn through their own personal experiences. And this leads to a great deal of chaos, confusion and disorder, of "trial and error", and of conflict and disharmonies, reflected as *war* in the world and *illness* in the individual. We are still in that period but now realize that we must continue growing up and evolving and that we need to transcend it if we wish to survive and thrive in the new century.

It is at this stage that *science* and the *scientific method* emerge and gradually supplant religion as the *via regia* to truth and reality. As it could be expected, given the fundamental perspective and set of assumptions of the West (Europe) at that time, the scientific method replaced tradition and authority with direct personal observation and experience. This greatly restricted what we call "reality" and "scientific truth" but it made that "restricted reality" much more meaningful and alive as it was grounded in direct personal experience. Thus the compendium of human knowledge that existed up to that time and which was integrated by religion broke down. The three essential fields of human study, *theology* (the study of God), *anthropology* (the study of man) and *cosmology* (the study of the universe) were redefined and splintered as was the discipline that studied their relationship and human significance, philosophy.

Cosmology became the natural or physical sciences, anthropology, the social or human sciences, and theology became more and more anemic and lost its social status and predominance. The fundamental perspective that gave a global vision of human knowledge and meaning underwent a major transformation and "fall". It became increasingly more worldly and secular, emphasizing the horizontal dimension and thus severing itself from the vertical dimension that began to slowly "fade away", being relegated to the realm of poetry, myth, and superstition. This in turn, led directly to materialism, rationalism, reductionism, egoism and hedonism which culminated in skepticism, cynicism, anomie, anxiety, alienation and depression. At the end of the 20th century and the beginning of the 21st century, this led to a major human crisis of increased confusion (both cognitive and moral), violence, demoralization, and destruction of our ecosystems and thus of the very foundation of life on earth, not to mention a health crisis.

Man found himself alone and alienated in the universe that was perceived as increasingly indifferent or hostile and overwhelmed by forces that were much bigger than he was and that he could neither understand nor control. Random chance replaced divine providence and universal law just as everything now depended upon what human beings did or did not do as there were no higher Beings to guide, inspire and heal them. Impotent and powerless, man began to feel that life was neither meaningful nor worthwhile and thus sought to escape reality via various addictions (alcohol, drugs, sex, or even work). The much larger panorama of Life in the spiritual and invisible worlds as well as in the material and visible world was reduced to *life in this world* which did not make much sense, seemed arbitrary and capricious to the extreme, and ruled by "luck" which abrogated any meaning and significance given to one's efforts and sacrifices. The survival of the fittest, might is right, physical force and violence, cunning, and power became the ultimate values. Such was the cosmos created by an adolescent humanity.

This obviously led to a growing crisis and sense of malaise, to the corruption and disenchantment with all social institutions: religion, government, the economy, education, the family health-care and even science itself which are now reaching their peak. This, in turn, led people to look for new solutions and to question what had happened, why we found ourselves in our present situation and what could be done about it. Towards the end of the second half of the 20th century, a major shift began to occur, focusing our attention upon all areas that could offer the promise of a solution, including Eastern and Western religions, esoteric and spiritual schools, transpersonal psychology, psychotherapy and personal growth. More and more people, including renowned scholars and scientists, began to realize that we had, indeed, "conquered the world" but "lost our soul" in the process (that is, a sense of meaning, purpose and *joie de vivre* that would make life worth-while and motivate us . . . in spite of its difficulties and sufferings).

With this state of affairs began the shift back from the horizontal to the vertical dimension with the realization that we needed to get out of the "black box" of reason and the senses that provided the cornerstone of science up to that point, to include *higher laws, energies, and faculties*. At the same time as human consciousness kept on growing and expanding, great souls and gifted children began to incarnate in our world to once again providing the inspiration and guidelines that are necessary for us to take our next "step" in evolution and to cope with the growing quantitative and qualitative challenges thrown to the human spirit. What people, who became interested in and started researching the more holistic and global approach that recognizes and integrates the spiritual dimension, discovered and concluded is, briefly, the following:

1. There are two kinds of knowledge: cognitive, mental and cerebral knowledge which is an *intellectual knowledge* about something and *experiential, direct knowledge* of something. The first comes essentially through our head psychospiritual center, involves thinking where there is a separate subject and an object, and is unable to move from the finite to the infinite and from the temporal to the eternal. The second comes essentially through our heart center, involves feeling where subject

and object fuse and become (at least temporarily) one, and which is able to progressively include the infinite and the eternal. Our Western civilization has become far too mental and cerebral, emphasizing knowledge and power over love and affection with the result that we have cut ourselves off from spiritual knowledge and wisdom to acquire an ever-proliferating scientific empirical knowledge. Now we must invert direction go through a *metanoia*: awaken our heart center and give priority to feeling and intuition over thinking and willing. A final implication of this is the fact that that while intellectual knowledge does not require a *specific life-style* (just the training and use of the mind) experiential, empathic knowledge certainly does and cannot be achieved without it! And thus we will no choice but to go back to a more balanced, healthy, and moral life.

2. Just as we have overemphasized having over being so we have also privileged analysis over synthesis. Thus now we need to go back to a proper integration and interconnection between the various fields of knowledge that we have acquired—to *synthesis*. We also need to realize that what is *alive* is qualitatively very different than what is *dead*, just like what is interacting with other systems is qualitatively different from what is isolated. Thus we need to take what is alive, what is interacting, and what is healthy and mature as our frame of reference rather than what is inert, isolated, and sick. While this is particularly important in health-care, it is also important in all other areas of life. In simple words, it means to take Saints, Sages, and spiritually awakened persons as our "models" or "point of reference" rather than sick or normal persons.

3. An important corollary of the first two points is that the time has come, as the need is great, for drawing from and relating *all important areas and disciplines of human knowledge*: religion and spirituality, psychology and biology, sociology and anthropology, and philosophy in particular. Most likely, this will require a new Renaissance in human knowledge and life, which this time will be a *spiritual one*! This transformation and rebirth will essentially be based upon an expansion, deepening and heightening, of our human consciousness as our evolution continues at this level; it will affect all areas of human knowledge and, therefore, all social institutions—changing our perception, definition and reaction of our human experiences.

4. A most important point, perhaps the distinctive characteristic of this *metanoia*, will be a major effort of introversion and supraversion: rather than focusing upon the world and the physical dimension to better know and control them, we will now refocus our attention and consciousness upon the microcosm of our own being and consciousness, thrusting towards *spiritual consciousness*. This implies a great deal of personal work and meditation as well as a proper understanding of the language

of the sacred traditions: symbolic and analogical language, whereby all symbols, archetypes, myths and rites are meditated upon and translated in terms of the *microcosm*, of our own nature and consciousness.

5. A proper understanding and integration of the male and female polarities, of human effort and divine grace, will be essential. For there are certain things that depend on us and others not, there are things that we must do because if we don't no one else will do it for us and they will remain undone . . . with our evolution being blocked! But there are also things that we cannot do and which only grace, or higher energies, can do for us. To be able to discern between the two and to have the intuition to gage, in different moments and circumstances, what we *can and should do* and what we *cannot do* will thus truly be essential just as it will be essential to remain humble, receptive, and open rather than falling prey to the stumbling block of pride, arrogance, and the assumption that we have the final definitive truth and that it is our duty or mission to impose it on others!

6. An overall and dynamic or growing and emerging understanding of human nature, human evolution, and human destiny, together with a holistic model of the psyche (of the nature, structure and functions of human consciousness) will also be crucial for this endeavor . . . as a proper theoretical underpinning for a "new encyclopedia" or compendium of human knowledge. For if people are going to be motivated and decide to act, they must know *why they are doing* what they are doing and *where* this will lead. The days of living in an *unconscious way,* being driven by inner desires and yearnings that we do not understand very well or being tossed here and there by external seductions, are over! We can no longer afford to do so as the consequences become more and more evident and catastrophic for ourselves, for others and for the world. Thus we must learn to live in a *conscious way*—know what we are doing, why, how, and where it will lead us to.

7. A final but most important point is that we have no choice but to discover and integrate the *vertical dimension*, the inner qualitative aspect of our lives that we have collectively and culturally neglected in the West for about 500 years. The 21st century will **be spiritual . . . or will not be** . . . thus we must direct our attention and efforts from the material and outer dimension to the spiritual and inner dimension. This implies activating our intuition, awakening our spiritual consciousness, and moving to a higher level of consciousness and being.

This tremendous transformation and redefinition of ourselves, of reality, of truth, and of what is truly worth-while will, unquestionably, affect not only ourselves and our consciousness (way of perceiving, defining, and reacting to outer and inner events). It will also affect *all of our social institutions*, leading to major revisions and restructuring in government, the economy, education, healthcare, the family . . . and religion! Religion has always existed and will always exist, in one form or another, in that human beings are truly *homo religiosus*, religious beings. The word "religion", in fact, comes from the Latin *religere, religare*, which means "to unite or to bind back" . . . first man with the various parts and aspects of his being and consciousness; but then also with God, the Ultimate Reality, with Nature, the physical world, and with each other.

The two most powerful forces and "guide-lines" or "frame of reference" for human beings are *religion* and *science*, religion in his childhood, science in his adolescence. Thus we could rightly ask ourselves, "What will these be in his adulthood"? I would suggest that religion, science and philosophyl/literature will be integrated in a higher synthesis woven around the *spiritual dimension* and with spiritual consciousness as its prerequisite! This new "synthesis" will also have to integrate the cognitive, the affective, and the conative dimensions with dynamic feed-back loops between them and is likely to culminate in the emergence of *spiritual science*.

In other words, it will have to link, in a dynamic, evolving process, *knowledge* (the head), *love* (the heart) and *will* (creativity and action in the world). For this to take place, we need to raise our level of consciousness, achieve spiritual consciousness, and then proceed to create a new cosmos out of chaos, both at the inner level (our psyche and consciousness) and at the outer level (the world and society). Now what can really help us to do so, in a simple, practical, essential, and effective way? Obviously Life itself, with all of its experiences and opportunities, but also our conscience and intuition, and its fruits: religion, science, and philosophy!

Here, my basic assumption is quite simple and clear: religion does have the answer to the most profound and universal human problems (in general) and to human suffering and salvation (in particular). But a most important distinction must be drawn here: it is not the "letter", the outer or "exoteric" aspects of religion but, rather, the "spirit", the inner or "esoteric" aspects of religion that can provide us with those answers. In other words, it is not the "religion of the people and the clerks" but the "religion of the Saints and Sages" that can do so! What religion, all authentic religions, have in fact done and are still doing is to carry forward through the centuries and to transmit *great mysteries* and *treasures* until such time as more and more human beings will be mature enough and have realized the necessary level of consciousness and being to properly "decipher" or interpret them and to put them to work in their lives, to incarnate them!

To my mind this time is NOW and the people who can do so are YOU! Perhaps the two most important "hermeneutic or explanatory keys" here are the analogies between the microcosm and the macrocosm and the proper understanding of the language of religion, poetry and the sacred traditions: symbolism, myths, archetypes and parables! It is also the Sacred Scriptures together with the oral tradition of the Church and the inspiration of the Holy Spirit which, today, I would call the **spiritual tradition**: the *Philosophia Perennis*, the *Hagia Sophia* or the *Primordial Tradition*!

To be able to access, understand and utilize properly, these mysteries and treasures, and for religion to experience its own "Renaissance" in the 21st century so that it will be in "consonance and resonance" with our present level of consciousness and evolution, we must raise and debate the following questions (for this is that will make it, once again, one of the most important and powerful forces for good, both for the individual and for society):

1. Can religion still remain a truly vital, living, and meaningful for in the 21st century? And, if so, how?
2. What are the "exoteric" and the "esoteric" aspects of religion, its "letter" and its "spirit"? And why do all religions and spiritual traditions always embody these two vital aspects?
3. Why is the connection between the "exoteric" and "esoteric" aspects of religion, its "letter", or outer aspect, and its "spirit", or inner aspect, so important today?
4. What are religion and spirituality in their essence? And what is their relationship to each other?
5. Is religion truly essential for "salvation" or not? And what is "salvation" anyway?
6. What is the meaning of "salvation" and "enlightenment" for the 21st century? What can they do for us? How can we achieve them and what is the price we must pay for doing so?
7. What is the role of the clergy and what are the clergy's *distinctive* contributions if any?
8. Why are a proper understanding of the "human sky-scraper" and of the nature and dynamics of language truly fundamental for a proper understanding and embodiment of both religion and spirituality in today's world?
9. Why are all human institutions, including religion, education and healthcare, "degenerating" and "crumbling" at this historical juncture and point in human evolution? For this is what is causing a true "crisis of trust" in today's world with disastrous results for "peace in the world" and "genuine health" in the individual.
10. What is the one truly fundamental factor that can help us understand and live through our present world-wide and multidimensional transformational crisis?

There are, of course, other related questions and questions that will emerge as we engage in this journey, but the foregoing are the core questions that I propose we look at and reflect upon together. I will be making some suggestions and share with you my own answers to the above. But this not as "the definitive answers" but rather as a "model" with a set of tools for *you* to come up with your *own personal answers*! For in the 21ˢᵗ century, in the period when humankind will reach its adulthood, there can be no ready-made and standardized answers, there can be only *personally lived and incarnated* answers!

As we already saw, the etymological meaning of the word "religion" is quite simple and clear: it means *to unite* or to *bind back* (and as such, etymologically speaking, it means the same thing as the word "yoga" or "psychosynthesis"). But to unite and bind back what? Briefly put, I would suggest what exists within ourselves, the microcosm, then ourselves with what exists outside of ourselves, the macrocosm (or God, Humanity, and Nature). I would also say to unite the microcosm with the macrocosm: the inner and outer dimension of reality; spirit and matter, and the male and female polarities.

As such, religion is always and can only be a *means* to an end and never an *end* in itself (which would make it an "idol" and thus defeat its very purpose!). The "end" here is spirituality which we will look at and define later on. Thus, it is most important not to confuse religion with spirituality (the means with the end) and to understand properly their respective natures, dynamics, functions, and objectives . . . if we wish to establish a right relationship with them that is in sync with the 21ˢᵗ century.

While there are *many* valid, authentic religions (which we briefly looked at and tried to describe in the first part of this work) that vary with the culture, the level of consciousness and being of the people who receive them and live them, there is but *one spirituality*! At the highest level and with perhaps an "Eastern" and a "Western" expression and manifestation, spirituality is fundamentally one as we are one! This means that, at its best, religion leads to, promotes, and accelerates the growth and expression of spirituality, while, at its worst, it can hinder, retard or distort spirituality.

Thus, religion is truly a mystery and a paradox for it has been responsible for bringing about the best and the worst in human nature and behavior! Some say that religion is, basically, quite simple and rational and that it can be understood and lived by all human beings, while others contend that it is quite complex and suprarational so that it can only be properly understood and lived by those who have activated their intuition and awakened their spiritual consciousness (Saints, Sages, Prophets and Initiates).

Religion as it is known and practiced, however, is generally institutionalized, rationalized and presented and explained in an intellectual or cognitive form. Genuine spirituality, on the other hand, can only be very personal, being grounded upon *direct personal observations and experiences*. Thus, religion can be taught in schools and described in books, while spirituality cannot as it must be personally lived and experienced. Human beings, teachers and masters, can transmit and propagate religion but not spirituality. For authentic spirituality can only come, ultimately, from the Self, from the divine spark within, from the Lord.

While religion is very important and can present a "picture", a "blue-print" or a "promise" of spirituality, it cannot confer genuine spirituality upon another human being . . . who must "achieve it"! Thus religion can be turned into an "idol", into a very destructive force, which can negate its very own highest purpose; the "letter" in other words, can kill the "spirit". Religion, therefore, is **not necessary for salvation**. What is necessary is **love**, both in its vertical expression as the "love of God" (or prayer) and in its horizontal expression as the "love of our fellow human beings" (or service), while the cement that unites and makes possible both is **love** and **faith.** Properly understood and lived, religion can *greatly accelerate our own development and evolution* and lead to the birth of genuine spiritual consciousness. But, misunderstood and misapplied, it can also do the very opposite as it has done in certain places and in different historical times.

It is quite difficult to define and conceptualize "spirituality" in that it is, preeminently a personal, direct, and lived experience. Still, we can attempt to gain some cognitive closure as far as its nature, dynamics and expressions are concerned. Thus, I would personally define spirituality as

> *"All those levels of consciousness that lie above and beyond*
> *sensory, emotional, and mental consciousness".*

When genuine spiritual consciousness is born and manifests itself in the consciousness and life of a person, it can be characterized by the following basic characteristics that are both unmistakable and distinctive. These are:

1. *The solution of the Riddle of the Sphinx:* That is for a person to be able to finally be able to answer the questions: "Who am I" (the problem of identity)? "Where do I come from" (the problem of origins)? "Where am I going" (the problem of destiny)? And, most important, "What have I come to do in this world" (the problem of "duty" or vocation)?
    As our essential being is of spiritual nature and origin, it is only when we truly develop our spiritual consciousness that we can properly understand who we are, what God is, and what we have come to do in this world; that is, answer the most fundamental questions of Life!

2. *The final overcoming of the primordial fear of death and dying.* For most people and for all those who have not awakened their spiritual consciousness, the fear of death and dying is, unquestionably, the most profound and universal fear and insecurity they have. This is truly the core "root" or "source" for all the other fears, insecurities, and negative

emotions. Through spiritual consciousness, we become aware of the fact (in a direct experiential way) that we are *immortal beings*, that Life has no beginning and no end, and thus that we cannot and will not "die" with our body (which has to die)!

3. *The tapping of two basic sources of energy or Life.* It is well-known that fear and insecurity burn up a great deal of energy and vitality. Hence, shedding one of the greatest sources of fear and insecurity cannot fail to also *liberate a great deal of psychic energy* which can then be utilized for other purposes. Not only, when we awaken and express our spiritual consciousness we can also access *spiritual energies* that can flow and be transformed into psychic and physical ones!

4. *The development of a true joie de vivre.* Last but not least, when we awaken our spiritual consciousness, we can then develop a spontaneous and profound understanding, appreciation of, and gratefulness for the immense privilege of living in, and experiencing the manifold "adventures" of Life in the physical world of Creation.

While there are other, more technical and detailed features and consequences of awakening one's spiritual consciousness (such as apprehending ourselves and reality as a trinity, accessing genuine inspiration and guidance, and discovering the spiritual Self, or divine spark: an inexhaustible and living Source of Life, Love, and Wisdom), the above should suffice to make our point. In essence, spiritual consciousness enables us to finally "awaken" and empowers us to "live fully and consciously". It does this by enabling us to find truly satisfactory answers to the most important questions of life: who we are, what are the world and Life, why we were born in this world, who is God really and what does He expect from us—what is true and what is false, what is good and what is bad for us!

Before that pivotal event that takes us from "childhood" into "adulthood", we were either "asleep", "dead" or as yet "unborn"; that is *unconscious* of what is truly essential! This is the reason why spiritual awakening is so important and why Jesus said many times, "seek ye first the Kingdom of God (read "spiritual consciousness") and all "these things" shall be added unto you" (you will then know and be able to do what is most important). The central thesis of this work and of my own approach to religion is quite simple and clear: For religion to survive and thrive in the 21st century (as a truly meaningful and alive force), it must rediscover its "esoteric" dimension and establish a dynamic and meaningful relationship between the "letter" and the "spirit" (the exoteric and the esoteric aspects)!

Every religion, spiritual and metaphysical tradition, as well as most academic fields, necessarily have "exoteric" and "esoteric" aspects. The reason for this is quite simple: people who live in this world do not all function on the same level of consciousness and being! I have attempted to present and elucidate this, in a rational and comprehensive way, through the basic insight of the "human sky-scraper" and the analogy of the "vertical axis of consciousness". As human beings do not all function on the same level of consciousness and evolution, they do not perceive, define, and react to the same phenomenon in the same way. Truth and Reality are thus, unquestionably, direct functions of the level of consciousness, being, and evolution of a person! By changing our level of consciousness, we literally change the reality that we perceive and live. And this is the deeper foundation for the need and importance of genuine forms of "conversion" or *metanoia*.

The word "exoteric" means external, given to all, not requiring a special preparation: purification, consecration, or spiritual gifts. It also involves a rational, cognitive, or intellectual approach to any subject that can thus be experienced, put into words, and transmitted to others. Finally, it also implies "lower levels of consciousness and being" that are accessible to all people as it is the "lower common denominator". The word "esoteric", on the other hand, means internal, given to the few, and requiring a special preparation: purification, consecration, and spiritual gifts. Essentially, it involves a *direct, personal observation or experience* of a given subject which can thus not be adequately expressed in words or taught to others as it implies higher levels of consciousness and being.

The "exoteric" aspect comes, essentially, from our personality, our human self or ego, whereas the "esoteric" aspect can only come, ultimately, from the spiritual Self, from the divine spark. Both aspects are, obviously, important and complementary, the first constituting the "letter" of a given tradition while the second its "spirit". Today, at our present level of consciousness and evolution, it is essential that they be connected to each other . . . just like a picture is connected with the person, or the object, that it represents!

Every important entity that exists, including God, Man and the Universe, but also religion and other academic disciplines, can be conceived as being made up of a *body*, a *soul*, and a *spirit*. The "body" is simply the material object and the physical dimension or support for any given phenomenon. The "soul" is the meaning: the implications and applications that are given to that phenomenon. Finally, its "spirit" is the power and life that lie behind the living meaning and applications of that given phenomenon.

From this perspective, therefore, the "exoteric" aspects constitute the "body" of religion and some of its most obvious and "down-to-earth" meanings; whereas the "esoteric" aspects constitute the "soul" and "spirit" of religion—some of its deeper and higher meanings and the power and energies that these can evoke and set in motion. Another way of look at this could be the following: the "exoteric" aspects of religion deal with its more tangible and concrete "worldly" significance and applications, whereas the "esoteric" aspects lead one towards spirituality, toward the end or goal that this aspect of religion is presenting to its followers.

The central objective, or fundamental goal, of the "esoteric" perspective is to translate and interpret all the symbols (images, archetypes, and rituals) of a given tradition in terms of the *microcosm*, of each individual person! As such, it is rooted in the twin assumptions that a human being is, indeed, a microcosm of the macrocosm (a fractal or synthesis of all there is). According to this perspective, whatever exists *outside* of us also has a correspondence *inside* of us! If in the external world we find the trinity of God, Nature, and Humanity then we must also be able to find the corresponding aspect of this trinity within human nature, within our own self. This is the central "explanatory key" of the "esoteric" point of view as well as its central objective: to meditate and reflect so as to find the correspondence and applications of all historical events and external persons, as represented in symbols and archetypes, and to translate them and apply them to the microcosm.

Another, the second most important assumption of the "esoteric" perspective, is that the language of the sacred traditions, of religion, spirituality and poetry, is not the same as that of everyday speech and science and must thus be treated in a very different way. The words of everyday speech utilize "terms" that convey and elicit thoughts and feelings whereas the concepts of science convey and elicit only one thought, or denotation, with an empirical referents and no connotations. The language of the sacred traditions, on the other hand, utilizes *symbols* rather than words or concepts. Symbols are designed to activate our intuition in addition to conveying and eliciting thoughts and feelings. Thus, it constitutes truly a symbolic and analogical language that is dynamic, living and which is a function of our level of consciousness and being.

These symbols, images, archetypes, and rituals, therefore, have a multiplicity of meanings, implications and applications that will unveil and manifest themselves as a person transforms and raises her/his level of consciousness. In the Middle Ages, this was understood as monks and nuns practiced the *lectio divina* that is reading one page of the Bible and then reflecting and meditating upon it for a year . . . to discover its deeper theoretical implications and practical applications. Thus, until the Reformation, the Bible and Sacred Scriptures could not be read and understood properly by anyone as they would read a normal book or newspaper! They had to be properly "interpreted and decoded" by the clergy, as it were. Two were the basic factors that would greatly help the personal work of meditation and reflection: the oral tradition of the *Ecclesia* and the inspiration of the Holy Spirit . . . which blended into the *spiritual tradition* on different levels.

What this means, practically and concretely, is that one can use the same symbol, ritual or prayer, over and over again and, each time, discover *new meanings and applications* or correspondences that were not recognized before.

In fact, whenever a symbol, image, archetype or ritual, is used in a practical and living way, it should always be "unique" and bring forth something new and fresh! I am personally convinced that it was the tragic confusion between the language of everyday speech, the language of science, and the language of the sacred traditions, together with the literal and fanatical attitude on the part of some religious leaders and faithful, that brought about the controversies that pinned science against religion and that "fractured" our conception of reality in the process!

Thus, every word (some even say every letter and its numerical valence) every symbol, image, archetype, myth, and prayer has *innumerable* meanings; implications and applications that the serious postulant must discover, personalize and relate to his/her life. A fragment of this insight can be found in the ancient American practice to have a Bible available in every hotel room! Each day, upon waking up or going to sleep, the person staying there could open, at random, the Bible, read one page of it and translate it in such a way as to be meaningful and applicable to his/her life and particular situation.

Thus, each words, symbol, image, archetype, prayer, myth or ritual is a *treasure-house* of information and practical insights. The problem is that, being so, it is very personal and "unique" thus requiring that person to *do the work required* and discover his/her personal correspondences that apply to his/her unique situation. Obviously, there is also a general and universal meaning and set of correspondences, but these apply only at a high level of abstraction and must be "brought down" and "applied" in a unique fashion by each unique individual!

Ultimately and at the highest levels, "salvation" and "enlightenment" actually are and imply the same thing: the awakening and integration of spiritual consciousness with sensory, emotional, and mental consciousness. Once grace or spiritual energy, which manifests as light and fire, has descended upon us and "illuminated" our head and heart psychospiritual centers then, by degrees, we will be connected with the inexhaustible Source of Life, Love, and Wisdom that dwells at the deepest level of our being and at the highest level of our consciousness . . . and thus we will be able to find an meaningful and satisfying answer to our most basic questions, needs and aspirations. In particular, we will then be able to answer the "riddle of the Sphinx", what we came to do in this world.

On a lower and more practical level, however, "enlightenment" implies a transformation and elevation of our consciousness which enables us to "connect with" and draws upon our *superconscious*. "Salvation", on the other hand, implies being able to consciously realize our destiny, fulfill the purpose for which we incarnated, and thus being truly ALIVE, to live in a conscious way and as an adult! Generally speaking, it is the Oriental traditions that speak of "enlightenment" while the Western ones speak of "salvation". The East is primarily concerned with the problem of human suffering, how to understand it and extinguish it; how to free the soul from the wheel of Samsara (or reincarnation in the physical world) so that it can return to its true home (the spiritual worlds), break the hold of "Maya", or illusion, and access perfect happiness.

To do this, all the practical rituals of the Eastern traditions always move from the bottom up (awakening the Kundalini fire that dwells at the bottom of the spine to activate all the charkas and, eventually, reach the top of the head) thus bringing about illumination. Here, the essential work really means a transformation of consciousness and perception which is brought about by true knowledge. Thus, it is knowledge that frees us from ignorance and from the slavery and dominion of the senses and of the physical world.

In the West, "salvation" has acquired multiple meanings and implications, according to one's tradition and level of consciousness and being. Essentially, however, it refers to being able to discover one's true identity, origins, destiny and, in particular, one's *calling in this world* (or what one has come to accomplish in this world) which are the substance of what the "enigma of the Sphinx" is all about. Thus, it focuses upon understanding and being able to consciously collaborate in "God's Will and Plan" (which is our destiny and what we came to achieve in this world) and being able to incarnate and further it in a conscious and effective fashion. Here it is not only knowledge (the head psychospiritual center) that is involved but also and especially **love** (the heart center) and will (the shoulder centers).

In other words, knowledge, understanding, and awareness are simply not enough; one must also learn to love and to have faith, to be able to do and accomplish things in the material world. Salvation, therefore, means to know who and what one is, to be able to be one's self, and to consciously express one's self in the world. And this is what it means to become and adult rather than remaining a child or an adolescent—which is the plight of most human beings and, in particular, of those who have not yet achieved spiritual consciousness.

The role of the ordained clergy of any religion is to be the repositories and transmitters of the "letter" of revelation and to be *unconscious vehicles for divine grace,* or spiritual energies; it is *to bless* (raise the consciousness and hence *heal* and *enlighten*) both people and the world. The clergy generally assumes diverse roles that can also be fulfilled by professional persons: that of a social worker, of a psychotherapist and counselor, that of a friend and advocate, etc. But the truly distinctive function of an ordained clergy person is that of being able to *bless others,* i.e. to bring down, transform, and project spiritual energies and frequencies. Through ordination, the energy bodies and the psychospiritual centers of the clergy-to-be are affected and conditioned in such a way that he or she can now become an unconscious vehicle or instrument for such energies and bring them down from the higher planes to manifest in this world. This qualification and distinction is most important, for both clergy and laity, to become and to remember *who they really are* so as to make the most of this treasure of the spiritual tradition.

When people (both clergy and faithful) will have reached a higher level of consciousness and being and activated their psychospiritual center, they will be able to see or, at least, *feel*, this blessing. Then "blessing" (others and the world) will become a true art and science, and bring many benefits to humanity and to the world. Experiments could be devised to train and sensitize people to their higher energies and frequencies and various technologies could be developed and used to render "empirical" and make manifest these higher energies which are conveyed by blessings. Here, I am thinking of Kirlian photography and Aura imaging in particular. The energies and frequencies that are channeled through blessings can be used for many different purposes. For example, to heal and activate one's immune and hormonal systems, for raising a person's level of consciousness and thus bringing about a genuine conversion, and to activate and integrate one's psyche so that he can now do spiritual work and obtain tangible results.

Most people anywhere in the world would concur that, today, human civilization is falling; that living conditions in the world are not getting better, they are getting worse, and that life is becoming more and more complex, difficult, confusing and thus stressful. Thus, there is little doubt that we are, slowly but inexorably, heading for a major *planetary crisis*. Some call it the Apocalypse, others the Kali Yuga, or simply the fall of civilization and degeneration. I like to call it the "crisis of adolescence" which will culminate in a major "maturity exam". Thus we can see that the great social institutions that have always been the basic "scaffolding" or "underpinnings" of both individuals and societies, namely the major social institutions (religion, education, government, healthcare, the family, etc.) are literally "crumbling" and can no longer be trusted and thus relied upon. And this is particularly true of religion, medicine and education!

This situation is what I like to call the "corruption of the experts" or the "crisis of trust", the heart of which is: "whom can I really trust and on what level can I trust them or not?" That this state of affairs exists today and is actually intensifying, few people would deny! The central point, however, is not that it is occurring but *why*? Is this the design of the Higher Powers, a consequence of our own values and choices, or mistakes (or both)? Or is it simply because of "blind chance" and random evolution? Different people, on different levels of consciousness, would naturally give different and even contradictory explanations. To my mind, however, nothing, and I mean *absolutely nothing*, ever happens by chance or without a deeper meaning and purpose. Thus, for me, this "sorry state of affairs" is definitely part of God's Plan or of our destiny . . . which we have created to a large extent! More specifically, it corresponds perfectly with the "adolescent" stage of evolution in which we now find ourselves.

The central message and challenge, brought about by this situation, is quite clear and simple, albeit far from easy to live! It is that now each person must look *within himself/herself* rather than at the world! That each person is now called to become a conscious, responsible, and autonomous person, that is an *adult* . . . rather than remaining a child or an adolescent who needs external points of reference and guidance! Having reached the threshold of the awakening of spiritual consciousness, a person must, necessarily, learn to be "true to himself", to be "inwardly" rather than "outwardly" guided, and thus to become independent of all external structures and points of reference. This process is certainly not easy or without risks, but it is indispensable and definitely worthwhile! And for this to happen, the great social institutions, the experts, the parents, teachers and external authorities, or "points of reference" must, necessarily, recede into the background and fade away . . .

The one factor that is truly essential, the "Archimedean fulcrum" to properly understand religion and spirituality in this perspective is the transformation and expansion of human consciousness from a lower to a higher level! Just like the physical universe is "growing" and expanding, so human consciousness is also growing, experimenting, transforming and expanding! This leads to quantitative and qualitative transformations of our knowledge and understanding, of our sensibilities and feelings, and of our creative energies . . . which can be very rationally and coherently explained by the insight of the "human sky-scraper" and the analogy of the vertical axis of consciousness.

Reality and truth are, indeed, a function of the level of consciousness, being, and evolution of the person apprehending them, and these change and transform themselves as we expand or contract the former. Another crucial element and insight of my philosophy of life (and for explaining what we are presently witnessing and experiencing) is the fact that we are presently in the midst of a very important transformation and expansion of our consciousness: we are changing levels or "floors of the human sky-scraper"! Both individually and collectively, we are moving from one floor to a higher floor on the vertical axis of consciousness—we are passing, in other words, from adolescence into adulthood, from the rule of the personality to that of the soul!

And this does, indeed, constitute a very major "passage" and "metamorphosis", involving great pressures and tensions, anxieties and insecurities, but also magnificent promises and rewards! As the ancient Sages used to say, "in order to become Man or Woman (an adult) a person must be able to answer the "riddle of the Sphinx" and thus cope with the problems of identity, origins, destiny, and "duty" or vocation. This, in turn, presupposes the activation of the intuition and the awakening of spiritual consciousness.

From an evolutionary standpoint, Life now demands that we get in touch with, and consciously harmonize, the male and female polarities of our consciousness and being. This, in turn, has an important prerequisite: that we activate our intuition and learn how to use it in our daily lives. For a quite a while now, I have become convinced, and this conviction is increasing with the passage of time, that within a few years (3, 5, 10, 15 years, I am not sure) if a person has not gotten in touch with and activated her intuition, she will functionally be in the same situation as an illiterate person is today! That is, that person will be lost and cut adrift on the "sea of life" and depending on so called "experts" or "external points of reference" which may no longer be there or, in any case, which may no longer be trusted!

In simpler words, Life now demands that we become conscious, autonomous, responsible beings that can *manifest spirit in matter* and that can consciously carry out their work and mission in the world. To truly discover and be able to draw upon that inexhaustible Source of Life, Love and Wisdom that we all have (the divine spark or spiritual Self), apparently the outer authorities and "frames of reference" must wither away . . .

One of the reasons why we are facing today so many paradoxes and contradictions, why we "have so much" and yet are "riddled with so many problems and unhappiness" is that, collectively speaking, we are *touching bottom*, we are reaching the nadir point wherein involution must turn to evolution. Until now, our civilization and culture, at least in the West, was secularizing itself, was becoming more horizontal, and was freeing itself from the "shackles of religion and custom", seeking greater "freedom" and self-expression by moving further away from the spirit to enmesh themselves deeper into the outer material world. Rationalization, reductionism, and empiricism were used to that end. Now, however, we must invert that tendency and move from matter back to spirit, move from having to being, and from an emphasis upon the male polarity to an emphasis on the female polarity, all the while keeping these polarities in proper balance.

When it comes to "theory and methodology" in approaching spirituality, these are relatively simple, provided one understands certain essential points which are the following: Spirituality is a state of being and consciousness that is the product of higher levels of consciousness than the normal, everyday ones. As such, it must be grounded upon a *direct personal observation or experience* of whatever we are concerned with. Being an immediate and direct experience and realization, it cannot be properly conceptualized and taught, rather, it must be *lived*!

Authentic religion always came out of such experiences lived by special, spiritually awakened persons. Then, what we know as religion became rationalized, codified, and dogmatized (i.e. scaled down to a humanly comprehensible level) by persons who are, usually, intellectuals and "ordinary persons" and not mystics . . . so that it can be understood and applied by "normal persons". This is where the "gap" and "difference" between the exoteric and esoteric aspects of religion spring from. Both aspects are necessary and connected with each other, but they certainly are not the same!

The heights and depths and many of the nuances and subtleties of the spiritual or mystical experience are thus "lost" by religion even though these can be retrieved by persons who have developed their spiritual consciousness and who can "cross" and "unite" the bridge between the "letter" and the "spirit' of that religion. In our world of duality where everything, without exception, can be **used or abused**, it is also a fact that religion (all religions) has produced both the best and the worst or human nature and experience. They have led many men and women to become enlightened, to become Saints, Sages, and Realized Human Beings; but they have also killed tortured, maimed, and persecuted people who did not agree with or who differed from their particular form of revelation (and its interpretation)—who did not obey or conform to their established dogmas.

Thus authentic religion must originate from and lead to *genuine spiritual experiences*, the purpose of which is to help people "reconnect" with the divine and understand God's Will and Plan for them. As such, it cannot be fully rationalized, dogmatized, or translated into human words; it can only be expressed in symbols, analogies, and metaphors . . . which must be interpreted and understood in different ways on different levels of consciousness and being. Hence, it should not be identified with established popular religion or confused with psychic powers or experiences.

As for "methodology", this, too, is quite simple and straightforward: religion (the means) and spirituality (the end) can either be approached or studied *intellectually*, by reading texts and their commentaries, or *experientially*, through one's direct vision and experience of the concerned phenomena and processes. Unfortunately, it is the first approach that is used, overwhelmingly, in the West and in their seminaries, theological schools, and courses on religion and spirituality!

Now it is one thing to be able to hear and read something which will then "awaken" something in your own being and consciousness, or "resonate" with your past experiences, and quite another to simply read something which is completely new and which does not resonate or evoke anything in your consciousness. To use an analogy, this is a little bit like the relationship that exists between a person and a picture of that person. The picture is not the person, but it evokes and reminds you of the person. If you know and have met that person in your life, the impact will be quite different than if you have never seen or actually met that person!

Using the profound analogy of the "Prodigal Son", so long as we were moving away from the "King's Palace and Realm" (the higher spiritual worlds), we focused more upon the picture. Now that we are returning to our "Father's Palace and Realm" (the higher spiritual worlds), we will once more have to distinguish between the two . . . and focus more and more upon the person! For a deeper understanding of the esoteric aspects of Christianity and the ability to translate the "letter" so as to arrive at the "spirit" of that tradition, I would refer the reader to my other works on this subject, *Divine Light and Fire, Divine Light and Love* (Element Books, 1992, 1994) *Prayer: the Royal Path of the Spiritual Tradition* and *The Spiritual Family in the 21st Century* (Xlibris, 2003, 2005).

Basic UN protocol or paradigm applied to religion and spirituality:

Central thesis: Without the esoteric aspect, the "spirit" of religion will not survive in the 21st century.

Fundamental objective or goal of this work: What constitutes the esoteric aspect of religion and how can we link it with the exoteric aspect?

Theory and methodology: Understand and learn how to apply the insight of the "human sky-scraper", the analogy of the "vertical axis of consciousness" and the of relationship between the microcosm and the macrocosm; also learn and apply symbolic analysis, theurgy, and consciousness transformation.

Concrete examples and illustrations: We can apply our prospective, theory and methodology, or "key of interpretation" to the symbols and archetypes of: *Extra Ecclesia nulla salus*, Jesus Christ, the Virgin Birth, the Sign of the Cross, etc. These are "models", or examples, that can then be applied to the other symbols, parables, and myths.

Practical applications: to the Church, Prayer, the Mass or Divine Liturgy, etc.

Core exercises: The functions of the psyche and the five basic "muscles of human con- sciousness". Learning how to work with symbols and archetypes, with ritual and theurgy. Learning how to consciously change our level of consciousness.

Central impact and core benefit: This perspective and the practical work it suggests will help you to transform and raise your consciousness, thus enabling you to know and understand more (head), to love and feel more (heart), and to have more creative energy, life force (shoulders), to express yourself better and become more alive.

Finally, I believe that we are also transforming and expanding our moral or ethical view-point. The old morality argued (in the dualistic fashion that characterizes most of our human experience in this world) that reward and punishment was the key to developing a viable "moral conscience". Society, religion and the criminal justice system told people what was right and what was wrong. They admonished them and rewarded them for doing what was "right" (i.e. expected of them) and they punished them when they violated society's basic norms and laws.

Having reached a certain level of consciousness and evolution, this approach is no longer viable as it seems to do violence to the "freedom of choice", or free-will" of a person which is his most important and sacred attribute. The new and emerging approach, instead, will tell people that they are *free to choose*, but that all choices have *consequences* that they will have to assume! Basically, it will say and tell people the following: "What do you really want? If you do this, here are the consequences and if you do that, here are the consequences! Which consequences do you want to assume and are you aware of them?" These "consequences" are not a "reward" or "punishment" for their behavior but an opportunity to discover themselves, life, the universe . . . and thus an opportunity to learn, grow, and evolve!

Thus, in conclusion and synthesis, reread carefully and meditate upon the present chapter, either in part or as a whole. Then, make a synopsis of its most important points and reflect upon the theoretical implications and the practical applications these may have for you and for your life today. Specifically:

1. What are religion and spirituality, and their relationship to each other, for you today?
2. What is your conception of "salvation" and "enlightenment" and what practical differences can these make in your life and being?
3. Is religion truly essential for "salvation" or not? Can religion remain a truly vital, living, and meaningful force in the 21st century as far as you are concerned. And, if so, how?
4. What are the exoteric and esoteric aspects of religion and their interrelationships to each other for you? Are these concepts meaningful and practical for you?
5. Why are a proper understanding of the "human sky-scraper" and of the "vertical axis of consciousness" so important? What insights can they contribute?
6. Why is a proper understanding and utilization of language, symbolic and analogical language in particular, so important for a proper relationship to religion and spirituality?
7. Do you see all or most social institutions (including religion) degenerating and "crumbling" at this historical juncture, thus creating a true "crisis of trust". If so, what do these mean to you and what can you do about it?
8. From your standpoint, what constitutes the one, truly pivotal factor to understand our present "period of transition" and the major and world-wide *qualitative crisis* we are presently living through? How can

one, meaningfully and practically, find hope, motivation and life (vital energy) in this situation?

9. As far as you are concerned, do the clergy (of any religion) still have a truly distinctive role and contribution to make?

10. What are the true nature and role of choice, values, and morality for you?

Last but not least:

- Are you able to find a way to make prayer and ritual (thus any religious service) truly come alive for you, vivify you, and recharge you . . . so that you will be self-motivated to continue and give time, attention, and energy to them?

- Have you ever really been confronted with and raised the "truly fundamental questions of Life": the riddle of the Sphinx, the nature and existence of God, the universe, life, and good and evil what is true and real and what is false and an illusion; of whether you should have a life-partner and how to choose that person; and of the kind of work that you should do for a living and for a vocation?

- Have you ever wondered about how to find a religion or a spiritual teacher that would truly be essential for you?

- Were you to die within a short period of time, what would you want to tell others and what would you want to leave behind?—what is truly essential for you?

- What are your present views and conceptions of life and death, health, illness, and healing, justice and injustice?

- What is the human condition? Why is it characterized by so many paradoxes and contradictions? Does it have a true meaning and end-purpose, an "intelligent design" for you? If so, how can you discover these?

- What are destiny, free-will, and grace for you at this time? Can you really make a difference in your life and in the world, and if so how? What depends on you and what does not depend on you in so far as your life and being are concerned, and how can you tell which is which?

- When nothing seems to work anymore, when you have tried everything and when "nothing works anymore", what can you do? What is your very last hope? How can you move from the horizontal to the vertical dimension?

Chapter II

THE CHURCH,
THE IMAGE OF HUMAN NATURE

Exploring and analyzing the symbol and archetype of the "Church", or Temple of God, as an image or reflection of human nature will provide an excellent "model" or "example" of the application of the spiritual perspective to a key symbol; of linking the exoteric and esoteric aspects of this "image" or the "letter" with the "spirit" which can then be applied, in the same way, to many other symbols and archetypes. Rather than merely hinting at possibilities and making a few practical suggestions, which is what I have done so far, with a number of sacred symbols and archetypes, I shall now provide you with a systematic and in-depth analysis which will begin to unveil some of the mysteries and treasures that are contained in this perspective and thus show you what can be done and how the spiritual perspective works.

Thus, this image and symbol will be "decoded" and "articulated" first through the basic insight of the analogy between the microcosm (man) and the macrocosm (the world and history). Then, we will utilize symbolic and analogical language to show some of its most important contemporary implications and applications. Finally, we will also suggest applying the "human sky-scraper" image and the analogy of the "vertical axis of consciousness" to show that this image and symbol, as all the others, contain multiple meanings, implications and applications, on different levels of consciousness and being. My basic thesis here and the evocative insight of the spiritual tradition is that any "temple of God", which is anchored in tradition and which respects sacred geometry, is really an *image or blue-print of human nature*, of the anatomy and physiology of our soul or energy-bodies with their psychospiritual centers. Thus, that when we enter a church or a temple, we simultaneously also *enter within ourselves*, we penetrate into our very own psyche!

120

From the very beginning of human history and all along the pilgrimage of humanity in the physical world of matter, man has been a religious being, that is a being who needs and longs to discover and consciously reunite with his Source, the essence of all that is and of Life, Love, and Wisdom in particular. As such, he has built countless temples, churches, and houses to the divine. In the spiritual or primordial tradition, it has always been a cardinal axiom that the "temple of God" should be built as a direct homologue or replica of human nature, which is also a homologue of God and of Creation; and this for many and diverse reasons.

Just as the physical body needs shelter from the elements and longs for a haven that he can call "home", so the spirit needs and finds a "home" in the soul, the soul in the psyche, and the psyche in the physical body! "As Above so Below", the law is the same on all dimensions and levels of being! Expressed in more mystical or "esoteric terms", *force* needs a *form* in order to manifest itself and unfold *consciousness*! And we know that the grand goal of evolution is to unfold and manifest consciousness, personal, individual consciousness wedded to universal, cosmic consciousness.

Thus, the Church, the Temple or Mosque, or by whatever name the dwelling of God is known, always (when it is linked with tradition, uses symbolic language, and respects sacred geometry) represents a *projection and objectification* (in stone or other physical materials) *of Man and his soul, the microcosm*. It describes, in very precise albeit analogical terms, the subtle, invisible and non-material *anatomy and physiology* of human nature. For he who has the proper "keys" or "decoder", any temple or even house (when built according to the teachings of tradition and sacred geometry) is an external blue-print of the human being made in the image of God.

Here, let us also bear in mind that we have a double mystery and treasure, the outer material one and the inner psychic one. Both are very important and complement each other and both must be properly understood and utilized . . . on different levels of consciousness and being. The outer temple or "material support" must be built in the right place, with the proper cosmo-telluric and angelic-spiritual energies; it must also be properly consecrated and then utilized just as it must contain the right symbolism and proportions . . . if it is to be used as an instrument to raise one's consciousness and accelerate one's evolution—as an instrument to bring and make *grace* (Light and spiritual energies and frequencies) available to us. The inner temple, which we carry with us wherever we go just like the snail carries its shell, contains a "labyrinth" which the symbolism and energies of the outer temple can help us to "walk through" so as to reach its center, the divine spark and spiritual consciousness.

Thus, for example, the Jewish Temple of Solomon, the Christian traditional church and the Muslim Mosque of Omar really represent an externalized picture and a blue print of man's psyche, of his psychic and spiritual anatomy and physiology, of his psychospiritual centers and their interrelationships, which are known as the

"Tree of Life", with their proper correspondences. Thus, when we enter into and stand in a classical Christian cathedral what we are really looking at is *ourselves* as created and made in the image of God and the Universe! What we see in stone, shape and color, are the inner and subtle levels which cannot be seen (at our present stage of evolution by most people) with the physical or psychological eyes alone. Yet this cathedral is not only *ourselves*, but also the union and point of encounter between the *microcosm and the macrocosm*. Thus, by meditating upon and entering into these magnificent "symphonies in stone", we can gain further understanding of ourselves and vivify our whole self-raise and transform our consciousness!

The living or Inner Church, the "Temple made in heaven not made not by human hands" is located within each and every human being. It includes specifically his psyche (human consciousness), his personality and his soul (or higher consciousness that includes spiritual consciousness). All outer temples and in some cultures even man's house are, in fact, an external symbol, a road-map, of the former. Depending on our level of consciousness and being, these can remain more opaque and veiled or they can begin to come alive, vivifying our intuition and imagination and providing orientation and proper direction in the spiritual worlds. So, never forget and always bear in mind that when you are entering a Church, you are really entering into the *Temple of your own being and consciousness!*

More specifically, you are entering into your own soul, or "energy-bodies", into your Tree of Life, their psychospiritual centers and the paths that connect them. This because whatever exists externally always corresponds to what exists internally . . . and vice versa. At the practical level, therefore, whatever the Priest does in the Church, you can do within yourself with the help of your "muscles of consciousness" linked with willing, thinking, feeling, creative imagination and intuition. Thus will the divine Light and the Spirit of God pour forth upon you, transform your consciousness, make you a temple of the Holy Spirit and activate the Christ within.

From the standpoint of this perspective, let us now continue and see what the Church building and its various symbols and rituals represent in the microcosm, how they can be entered into by the aspirant to the Mysteries, and what they might do for him/her (see illustrations 2.1: the Ancient and Modern Temple, 2.2: Man correlated with the Cross, 2.3: the Tree of Life, and 2.4 the Human Aura in the Tree of Life). In the physical plan of the Church, one can visualize a human being lying on his back with his arms outstretched and forming a Cross. Thus here we have a symbolic representation of the human body with its subtle vehicles of consciousness which represent his whole being. Thus, at the inner core of the Church's architecture and symbolism (described in the language of imagery and analogy . . . which is the language of the soul and of the Sages) we find a blue-print, a complete blue-print of man's psychic and spiritual anatomy and physiology, of his Tree of Life and "energy-bodies" and of their psychospiritual centers!

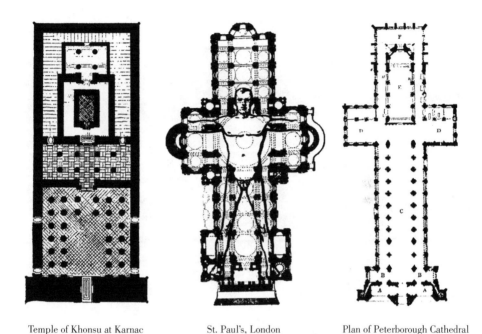

Temple of Khonsu at Karnac   St. Paul's, London   Plan of Peterborough Cathedral

Figure 2.1 The Ancient and the Modern Temple

An Egyptian Temple and two examples of Christian Cathedrals. These plans show the threefold division of the Human Temple. The plan of Peterborough Cathedral shows the average type of strictly cruciform cathedral, while the plan of St. Paul's shows the cruciform type adopted to the classical style of architecture; the circular feature at the crossing of the nave and transept have elements of Rosicrucian symbolism. The illustrations show Man to be the archetype of all Temples (George Plummer, *Rosicrucian Fundamentals*. New York: Flame Press, 1920 page 322.)

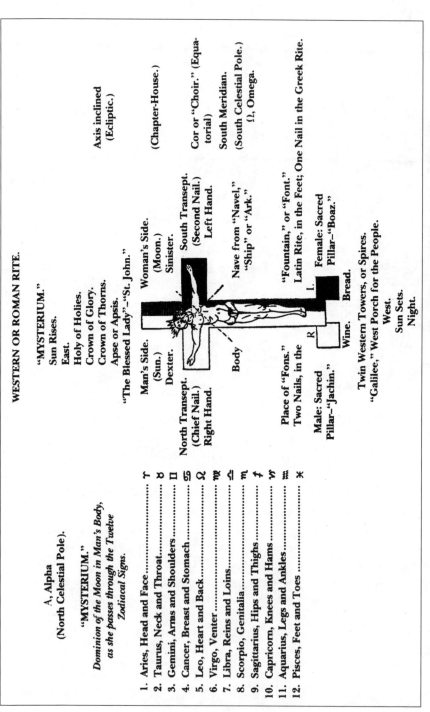

Figure 2.2 Chart showing man correlated to the cross and the cruciform type of church building (Hargrave Jennings, *The Rosicrucians* .)

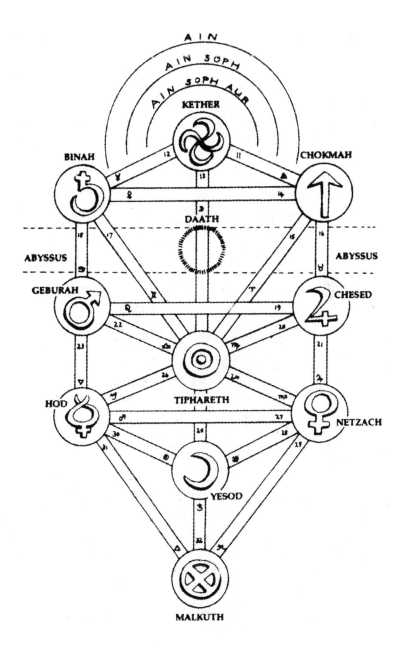

Figure 2.3   The Tree of Life

For further correspondences on the Tree of Life and the psychospiritual Centers, see Appendix B. (Melita Denning & Osborne Phillips, *The Sword and the Serpent*. Llewellyn Publications, 1975.)

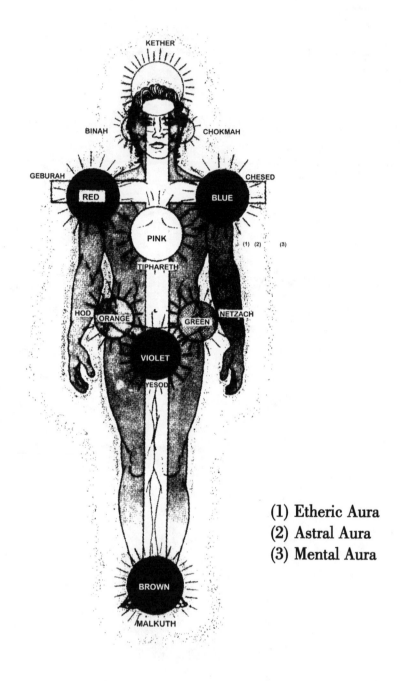

(1) Etheric Aura
(2) Astral Aura
(3) Mental Aura

Figure 2.4   The Human Aura in the Tree of Life

(Peter Roche de Coppens, *The Invisible Temple*. Llewellyn Publications, 1987.)

When a student of the Mysteries enters into a Church, or a physical temple, he is aware that he is entering, at the same time, into the temple of his own consciousness in order to focus upon inner events and psychospiritual processes. Thus, he leaves the external world in order to move from "profane space into sacred space", from "profane time into sacred time" and from "profane events into sacred events". Once he has entered into his own psyche, he makes an effort of introversion and concentration to leave behind all thoughts, emotions, and preoccupations about the external world to focus upon, completely and exclusively, the work and processes which he is about to begin and which involve an important aspect of the Great Work.

Thus, she is aware that the "place" in which she finds herself, the outer physical as well as the inner psychic temple of her psyche, is a *sacred space*. It is the place in which she finds herself in the presence of the living God, where divine Light, Fire, and Life are present and wherein she can become conscious of them. Thus, she becomes aware of the *axis mundi*, the "vertical axis of consciousness" that connects heaven and earth, which leads from the field of consciousness to the unconscious and the superconscious or, in another language, from "earth" to "hell" and to "heaven".

Finally, she is conscious of the fact that the work she is about to undertake is truly the most important work, the Great Work; that when she works upon herself and does internally what the priest does externally, she is able to contact the divine Light and Fire and thus to commune with her divine spark that will fill her being and her consciousness with Its Life, Love, and Wisdom. It is in this fashion that she can perfect herself in order to offer herself, her inner temple, more fully and consciously, to the spiritual Self so as to accomplish Its work and mission in this world.

There are several passages of the Bible (and of other sacred texts) which clearly and explicitly indicate that the physical temple, the church, or the "house of God", is but an external objectification of the "inner temple of the living God" which is the soul, the psyche, the personality and the body of a human being and, in particular, his *psyche*. In the Bible and the Christian tradition we find the following statements:

- "Jesus answered and said unto them, destroy this temple and in three days I will raise it up. Then said the Jews, forty and six years was this Temple in building and wilt thou rear it up in three days? But he spake of the *temple of his body*". (John 2:19-21)
- "Know ye not that *ye are the temple of God*, and that the Spirit of God dwelleth in you?" (I Cor. iii, 16)
- "If any man defile the temple of God, him shall God destroy; for the temple of God is holy, which *temple ye are*". (I Cor. iii, 17)

When looking upon the basic features and the architecture of religious temples throughout the ages, we find two distinguishing characteristics. They all have, more or less, the form of a cross and are subdivided into three basic parts. As a Sage stated:

- "The Egyptian Temple had its Outer Court or Court of the People; its Middle-chamber or Hypostyle Hall, and its Sanctum Sanctorum of Holy of the Holies into which none but the Hierophant entered. The Greek Temples has their Pro-Noas or Outer Court; the Naos or Cella, or Middle Chamber, and the Sanctuary or Holy of the Holies, containing the shrine or statue of the God or Goddess. The Hebraic Temple has its Outer Court or Place of the People, the Middle Chamber or Holy Place, and the Sanctum Sanctorum or Holy of the Holies to which similar reverence was paid by the High Priest. The Pyramid has its Unfinished Chamber on the Ground Floor; its Middle or "Queen's Chamber" and the Sanctum Sanctorum or "King's Chamber" although no King has ever been there. The Gothic Cathedrals besides being cruciform in plan, which is simply the Cosmic Man under the Sign of the cosmic Cross, have the Nave, or Place of the People, the Choir or Chancel for the Singers and the minor clergy, corresponding to the Middle Chamber, and the Sanctum Sanctorum or Holy of the Holies into which only the highest ecclesiastical dignitaries and the Celebrant and his assistants at the Alter enter" (George Winslow Plummer, *Rosicrucian Fundamentals*)

Man is made in the image and likeness of God therefore he is made in the form of a cross and a trinity. Hence the Church or Temple must also have the form of a cross and trinity. The cross is not only the symbol of the physical form of a human being but also the symbol of the Tree of Life which is the "skeleton" of the inner man, of his aura and psychospiritual centers. The trinity is not only the symbol of the structure of a human being (body, soul, and spirit) but also of the essential levels and expressions of his consciousness (conscious, unconscious, and superconscious; etheric astral, and mental body; knowledge, love, and life; will, thoughts, and emotions).

When the candidate enters into a church, he likewise enters into the temple of his consciousness. He enters at the bottom of the Cross at the level of Malkuth. There, through an effort of concentration and introversion, he leaves the world, the past and the future, as well as all of his mundane interests and concerns to focus his attention upon his inner anatomy and physiology. Then, he begins his ascension from the feet of the Cross, Malkuth, to Tiphereth, the heart center, to commune with the Light, Fire and Life descending from Kether.

The three pillars of the Tree of Life are represented by the aisles and naves of the church. The central aisle represents the pillar of Equilibrium, the left the pillar of Mercy and the right that of Severity. The door at the bottom of the church with its baptismal font symbolizes Malkuth; the first rows of chairs at the bottom of the church represent Yesod, the Altar Tiphereth, the heart center. The Dome above the altar or the rose window bringing light on the altar corresponds to Kether, the head center. The statues of the Virgin Mary and Saint Joseph, with their respective blue and red colored lights and garments, on the two side aisles, can be seen as reflecting Chesed and Geburah, the shoulder centers on the Pillars of Mercy and Severity. The rose windows on both sides of the church represent a composite mandala or symbols depicting Netzach and Hod, Chesed and Geburah, Chockmah and Binah respectively. Here we clearly have, represented in an analogical and symbolic fashion, the entire Qabalistic Tree of Life.

It is not only the church where one goes to pray and celebrate the Eucharist, and the inner work that one can do as preparation, that are important to determine the results one will obtain, it is also the place in which one chooses to sit in the church. The place we choose can have a profound impact upon our consciousness and its various functions which we will have to use to participate in the ceremonies being celebrated in the church. If we sit on the left side of the church not too far from the altar, that place corresponds on the Tree of Life to Netzach, the emotional center and lies on the path connecting Netzach and Tiphereth, the intuitive center of the heart which also corresponds to the altar. To choose to sit there means to work on the "opening of the heart" and the purification of one's emotions and connecting with one's divine spark through a more passionate, pure, and devoted love.

On the other hand, if I want to work on "opening the mind" and sharpening my intuition, I would sit on the right side of the church, a little lower than the above, in a space corresponding to Hod, the intellectual center. Rather than feeling passionately, I would then be concentrating upon thinking clearly, on meditating and discovering the various correspondences of the different aspects of the church and of the ritual which is being carried out and which I am interested in at that time. The important thing here is to decide what aspects of the Great Work you now want to focus upon and develop and then to experiment sitting in different parts of the church to see what happens and how you react to them as you change places. Because it is only *doing something* that will truly help us know it and master it!

In the churches and temples that have retained some of the ancient symbolism and correspondences of the holy Wisdom (in Christianity, the catholic traditions and the Orthodox Church in particular), we invariably find "veils" between the sanctuary with the altar and the main body of the Church; this can be a veil of cloth, an elaborate iconoclasia, or an enclosure. Likewise, at the other end of the church we can find a "veil" or an enclosure setting apart the choir, the crypt that may be there, or an enclosure with baptismal fonts or confessionals. These "veils" are there for a reason and can be compared to the "separations" that correspond, within human consciousness, to "breaks" between different levels of consciousness, for example between the conscious and the unconscious and the superconscious.

The various rose windows, paintings, statues, or other symbols one can find in a church have archetypal elements in them that help focus our consciousness upon certain psychospiritual centers, a certain level of consciousness, or a specific energy and frequency. Properly understood and utilized, these can help activate our intuition and open inspirational channels through a visualization and creative imagination process The four Elements are also prominently displayed and used in churches via the use of candles (Fire), incense and words (Air), wine and water (Water) and the bread and salt (Earth). In the Eucharist the four Elements are also present in the bread (Earth), wine (Water), the spoken words of the priest (Air) and the candle or candelabra (Fire).

The Priest with his assistants represent humanity and the psychic functions of the psyche (willing, thinking, feeling, imagination, and intuition) which all work together to bring through the divine Light, Fire, and Life of the divine spark and the Lord to the altar, the heart center. These are then given to the communicants so that they can, indeed, commune consciously with Christ and assimilate the divine Light and Fire of which the bread and wine are the vehicles. This spiritual Light and Fire can be felt and even seen by those who have acquired the necessary level of consciousness and sensitivity.

The members of the congregation represent the different cells of our body and the different subpersonalities of our psyche, which must be awakened spiritually and properly coordinated. When we go to Communion, we identify with the human self which must commune with the spiritual Self, represented by the priest. What this means, practically speaking, is that what the priest does at the altar, we must do in our heart center and consciousness. This because everything that takes place in the church is an *analogue* and *homologue* of what must take place in our aura and consciousness. As we approach the altar at the physical level, we should inwardly enter into our heart center which then "opens up" to the superconscious and the spiritual Self, represented by the sanctuary where the healing and vivifying Light will manifest.

Each prayer and petition mentioned by the Officiant can be repeated inwardly, focusing all of one's faith upon them (i.e. focusing his attention, thoughts, and emotions upon them). In this way, one will be using them in a *theurgic way* so that they will become conscious and operative, flooding one's consciousness and stirring to life many different states of consciousness, energies and vibrations . . . which will open a "channel" through which genuine intuition and spiritual consciousness will be able to manifest. Ideally, every word, formula and passage of the Liturgy should be meditated upon at home to discover some of its "treasures", inner meanings and correspondences. This can also be done a little before Mass or after it. During Mass, each word, phrase and gesture of the priest must resonate and fuse in one's being and consciousness so as to awaken new intuitions, thoughts, feelings, and energies. Finally, one must allow one's consciousness to fuse with them, to become them and to live them so that they can become "flesh" in us for it is then and only then that we and our lives *become them*, "living prayer" . . .

At the heart of worship lies the mystery of the heart of the worshiper and the heart of God because the heart is the true place where communion between the human and the divine can take place and because love is the truly essential quality and energy. Thus, it is not the "body" of the church or even of the ritual (the words and gestures of the priest) but their soul and spirit (their proper comprehension, interpretation, and application as well as the life and energy that lie behind them) that will make possible the psychospiritual transformation necessary to commune with God and to realize the Great Work! This is what the Divine Liturgy, the Mass, was designed to accomplish for all those who are ready to live consciously and to offer their whole heart, mind, and soul!

Likewise in the spiritual life, it is the temple that must serve the ritual and the ritual that must nourish the soul and bind it back with the spirit. The external church and ritual must serve the inner temple (the energy bodies, their psychospiritual centers and the sanctuary of the heart) and the inner ritual (the life and growth of consciousness). To be able to recognize and to live this is the Great Work and the "Great Work is a Great Love" and it is to this Work and Love that you are now all invited!

Chapter III

THE CHRISTMAS STORY, THE BIRTH
OF SPIRITUAL CONSCIOUSNESS

The next practical and concrete application of the spiritual perspective to a very well-known and universally commemorated event is that of the Christmas story in the Christian tradition. Remember that the central insights of the spiritual perspective and the esoteric interpretation of any religious event always refer to the microcosm, to *you:* to your consciousness, your life and your being! But you must do the work of interpretation and the correlation of the correspondences and associated symbols and this personal work, which only you can do and that is always a function of your level of consciousness and being. Thus, there will, necessarily, be multiple meanings, implications and applications that will change as you raise or lower your level of consciousness . . . which can be very different and even opposed.

Let us briefly review and bear in mind the most important characteristics of symbolic and analogical language which is the distinctive language of the sacred traditions. Symbols, images, and archetypes are:

- Multidimensional: they do not have one set of meanings that is pre-established and socially standardized but many sets of meanings and correspondences which, are, in fact, "open to infinity" as they are a function of our changing level of consciousness and being. Thus, they can "burst forth" with new, emergent meanings that can be directed and linked, analogically and homologically, with human nature, with the world and with unfolding expressions of human experience.
- They truly function as a "bridge", or link, between the known and the unknown, the knowable and the unknowable, and the conscious and the unconscious. As such they can both veil and unveil the truth,

or process, they represent and which they act as a media to convey to others.

- Each symbol, image or archetype must be "worked upon", "personalized", and "made to come alive" in the consciousness of the person using it. Hence, each symbol is truly like a *mine* which has to be individually "mined" to make it yield its treasures . . . just like a tree has to be fed, nurtured, and pruned to make it yield its fruit.

Thus no one can hand a symbol, an image or an archetype to another person "ready made" and "already worked out" for then it would automatically be transformed into a word or a concept and cease to be a genuine symbol. What this means is that each person has to become personally and actively involved with each symbol, rite or myth, and use all of the functions of his psyche to "make it come alive" in his own consciousness and being to "yield and reveal its treasures" which will vary and grow with the level of consciousness, the human experience, and the degree of maturity of the person who uses it.

Each symbol, moreover, has a three-fold nature: it has a *body* (the image or glyph), a *soul* (its growing, unfolding and emergent interpretation and application), and a *spirit* (the life or energies it is connected with and can release). What can be carried forward and transmitted from one generation to the next, from one person to the other, is its *body*. Its soul must be personally honed, nurtured and organically grown by the person who receives it in order to be lived and experienced. Finally, its spirit is the ultimate treasure, or gift, it will bestow upon those who have worked diligently with it and who are ready to receive it.

To pierce through the many veils of symbolism, on the different planes of being and levels of consciousness, we need to involve our whole being; that is, give it our whole attention and use the major functions of our psyche (willing, thinking, feeling, and imagination in particular) to decode its deeper meanings and correspondences. In a nutshell, we have to learn how to concentrate our attention upon it (willing), then to meditate on it (thinking), to visualize it (imagination), and to pour all of our feelings and emotions (devotion) into it so as to truly make it "come alive" and "reveal its mysteries" to us.

The four essential "muscles of human consciousness", or psychological processes associated with a given function of the psyche, are: *concentration*, linked with willing, *meditation* linked with thinking, *devotion* linked with feeling and *visualization* linked with imagination. Together these can activate the process of *invocation-evocation* linked with intuition which is fundamental for conscious and living prayer. Taking the Christmas story, its *dramatis personae* and its core symbols and archetypes, as a practical "laboratory" for the development of the core functions of the psyche and their associated "muscles", we can systematically practice and amplify:

- *Concentration* by focusing our attention upon one or more of these symbols,
- *Meditation* by reflecting upon and seeking associations that can reveal their deeper nature, correspondences, and associations.
- *Devotion* by pouring forth our love and emotions upon these symbols and
- *Visualization* by focusing upon one image or glyph for each core symbol or archetype used.

All of these are used for *praying* when we want our prayers to become conscious and alive. Finally, if used properly, these four "muscles" will culminate in and activate our *intuition*, the break-through of higher energies, frequencies and levels of consciousness through the process of *invocation-evocation*. Thus a whole curriculum of psychological development, leading to spiritual awakening and realization, can found in all of the major religious myths and their related symbols and archetypes.

Basically, there are three great realms of dimensions for the application of symbols, images, and archetypes with various connections, associations, and homologies between them. The first, obviously, is the literal, *historical, realm*: what happened in history; what were the occasion and the series of events through which this symbol or archetype entered tradition; who gave it to us and for what purpose? This could be viewed as "the body" of the symbol. The second is the analogical, *psychological realm*: the application of the symbol or the image to the microcosm, to human nature, to ourselves today and in the situation in which we find ourselves. This could be viewed as the "soul" of the symbol. The third is the metaphorical, *ontological realm* the application of the symbol to the macrocosm and getting in touch with the life and power that stand behind it which could be viewed as the "spirit" of the symbol.

The first realm or dimension is the one that is generally taught by religious and metaphysical traditions and which is best known to most people. The second realm or level constitutes what is generally known as the "Lesser Mysteries" and which is reserved for its initiates, for those who have trained and are ready for it. Finally, the third realm or level constitutes the Greater Mysteries and is reserved for its Adepts, for those who have reached the necessary level of consciousness and being to penetrate into its treasures and act as "instruments" or "channels" for the realization of God's Will and the divine Plan on earth.

Finally, symbols, images, and archetypes can also be used *theurgically* to create and bring about a new state of consciousness and being, and a new reality: the incarnation of a spiritual Power in Man and in the World. Here, it is the intuition with its twin processes of invocation and evocation that are being used. For let us remember that "psychic energy always follows thought and attention" and that the higher the level of consciousness, the intelligence and sensitivity, of a person and the greater will be the creative or destructive power of his thoughts and feelings.

For our present purposes, we shall direct our attention and analysis upon the story, or myth, of Christmas and its application to the microcosm, to our own self in the here and now. We shall use the *spiritual tradition* at the objective level and *meditation* and *reflection* at the subjective level to "decode" some of its inner, psychological and spiritual meanings, implications and applications. Please bear in mind that this constitutes but one set of meanings on one basic level of this profound set of symbols and myth which contains many others that are yet to be discovered and utilized. Thus it is suggested to you not as "its spiritual interpretation" but, rather, as *one interpretation* that is internally coherent, heuristically fertile, and which corresponds to an important level of consciousness and being that more and more people are now developing.

Thus Christmas is not something that simply happens of and by itself! Unless we fully participate in and co-create, within ourselves, its core events it will never take place. As the great mystic and poet Angelus Silesius once put it: "Though Christ a thousand times in Bethlehem be born and not within thyself, thy soul will be forlorn!" It is in this very simple and yet profound declaration that we find the essential esoteric key for the practical interpretation of this Event.

Christmas is but one of the three main Western and Christian holy days and myths, or composite symbols, the other two being Easter and Pentecost. While in its exoteric or outer aspect Christmas is the first major holy day or celebration, in its esoteric or inner aspect, it is the second, the middle and vital step between Pentecost and Easter with its final culmination in the Ascension. As such, it will provide a wonderful "model" or "point of reference" for the work that can be done with the others and with their equivalents in other religions.

When we apply Christmas to the microcosm, to our own consciousness and being and interpret it in terms of the Lesser Mysteries, the first thing that we notice is that this Event is not something that applies to the members of one religion only, to "Christians", but to all human beings regardless of their faith and religion or lack thereof! As such, it is truly a *human* and even a *cosmic* event that applies to humanity and to the world. The second point is that it pertains to and celebrates not so much something that happened in history, some 2,000 years ago, as something which is yet to happen in the future and in our *own soul and consciousness*. Lastly, we notice how far from being a "fait accompli" it is merely a vision, a glyph, or a prophecy of something which we can and must bring about by involving and developing all of our human and spiritual faculties . . . which will be complemented and completed by the free gift of the Pneuma and of our divine spark.

The very central meaning and the etymology of the word "Christmas" point directly to its deeper nature and function: *Christ-mas* means "making

Christ" or enabling Christ to be born in us so as to become a "Christed human being" . . . which is what happens when the Light of the divine spark descends upon and is born within our personality! The birth of Jesus of Nazareth 2000 years ago represents the image, the glyph, or universal archetype, of the *birth of our spiritual consciousness* within *our own soul*. It represents, symbolically and analogically, the conscious "connection", or proper alignment of our human self with the spiritual Self which will enables us to be reborn as spiritual beings, as children of God, in whom it is the Lord that will rule and manifest Himself.

As such this Event is one of the most important and crucial moments not only of this lifetime but of our entire evolution! It represents the culmination point and the cross-roads of a very long conscious and unconscious preparation towards and the entering into another level of consciousness and being. It is literally a "death" and "resurrection" and implies an "evolutionary leap" that is as great if not greater than our passage from the animal into the human realm. And as with the former, it takes place over a very long "incubationary" period of time and not instantly, at least in its preparation. Thus the story, or myth, of Jesus, with its many symbols and events, is truly a universal glyph and archetype of what is to occur to each and every one of us. As such it implies the working together, or "cooperation", of both human effort and divine grace. This myth or "blue-print" is like a map and the guiding light leading us by degrees to our long-coveted but dimly imagined destination—the descent of the Light and of God into our personality or human temple.

In the story or myth of Christmas, the great symbol and archetype of our spiritual initiation, we find certain persons, images and events which are:

- The Christ-child clothed with a white golden clothes or light.
- Mary and Joseph dressed in blue-white and red-white garments.
- The Immaculate Conception.
- The Magi and their three gifts: gold, myrrh and frankincense, and the shepherds.
- The manger into which Jesus is born.
- The star of the Savior.
- The animals, bull and donkey, who breathe upon Jesus.
- The Angels who sing "Glory to God in the highest and peace to men of good will".
- The Christmas Tree.
- Santa Claus or St. Nicholas.

All of these elements and components are found in the manger which is the mandala or composite glyph of the Christmas story. Seen through the optic of the Western spiritual tradition and of the Lesser Mysteries, they all apply to the *microcosm*, to the soul, consciousness and being, of *each one of us* and must accordingly be deciphered in this fashion. We can thus use the myth of Christmas and the central glyph of the manger as a "practical laboratory" to practice and develop the "muscles of our consciousness" (concentration, meditation, devotion, visualization, and invocation-evocation). They can also be used in a *theurgic fashion* to bring about the reality which they depict: the descent of the Light into our personality and our spiritual initiation.

Through meditating upon each one of them and their composite glyph we can discover the implications and applications of these symbols in the microcosm, in our own soul and consciousness. By their contemplation we can look upon and realize the "esoteric" or spiritual mysteries they might have for us at this point in our evolution. While through their theurgic use, we can realize and incarnate this process in our own consciousness and being—we can enable these images and work to become "flesh" in us. Seen from the standpoint of meditation and contemplation, here are some of the most important meanings, implications and applications, these symbols and images can have for us at this point in our evolution and at the level of consciousness and being we have achieved:

- The Christ child clothed with white and golden light represents the personification and manifestation of the divine spark that progressively incarnates Itself in our field of consciousness bringing Light, Fire and Life to our personality.
- Mary and Joseph represent, respectively, the essence and expression of the male and female polarities in their multiple manifestations. To give birth to anything—a child, an idea, an emotion, or spiritual consciousness—we need to work with both polarities. For God to be born in Man and to awaken spiritual consciousness, both polarities must work together in that the law is the same on all planes of creation. Here Mary represents *divine grace*, spiritual Light, or the spiritual energies that come down from above while Joseph represents *human effort* which works "from below" to reach for the stars. Joseph thus represents the human and psychological work which must be accomplished to "prepare the temple" while Mary symbolizes the spiritual answer to these efforts. Thus Joseph is the symbol of the promethean effort towards the superconscious and the spiritual Self while Mary embodies the epimethean response and the manifestation of the Light in our field of consciousness. In psychological terms, Joseph is associated with the *invocation* (the synthesis of concentration, meditation, devotion, and visualization) of the divine spark; whereas Mary is associated with *evocation* (the descent of the spiritual energies and the intuition) which revitalizes, transforms and amplifies our capacity to will, to think, to feel, and to visualize. In the legend of the Holy Grail Joseph represents the *spear* and Mary the *cup*. Mary is the "psychic or human matrix"

while Joseph represents the necessary human stimulus and invitation to bring down the spiritual energies so that they can manifest in our field of consciousness.

- The Immaculate Conception also contains multiple meanings, implications and applications on various levels of consciousness and being. Spiritually, it points to the fact that the soul of Jesus and of Mary are "immaculate conceptions", i.e. that they chose to freely incarnate in this world not for their own evolution or progress but for the world, *for others*. Their soul is free, without sin, karma or imperfections. We, on the other hand, and the overwhelming majority of human beings are born by necessity, "in sin" as it were, so as to grow, perfect ourselves and actualize our potentialities. It also indicates that the birth of God in our souls involves psychological and spiritual processes rather than physical ones. Thus, this "birth" is also an immaculate conception co-involving divine grace and human effort, the use of all of our "tools" and psychospiritual resources to which God will add His grace!

- The three Magi and their gifts symbolize, in the microcosm, the three royal functions of the psyche: thinking, feeling and willing which must work together to bring about spiritual initiation—the birth of spiritual consciousness. They must bring their archetypal gifts (or ontological qualities of both God and man) to the divine spark: Gold which represents consciousness and wisdom, Myrrh which represents the will and creative energies, and Frankincense which symbolizes love and feeling. For it is only when a human being can bring and offer his whole heart, mind, and will (i.e. all of his human love, knowledge, and energies) that these can then be vivified, purified, and transmuted by the Light into God's Wisdom, Love and Creative energies—into God's Will. What this means is that each one of us must bring his "gifts", the best of oneself, to the divine spark or the inner Christ; for it is with these energies and qualities that the divine can work in us and through which He can reveal and manifest Himself. Without this offer and sacrifice on our part, without offering our very self and consciousness as "channels" and "vehicles" for the Light, our knowledge, love, and will cannot be transformed and amplified by God Who would then be unable to manifest Himself consciously in our psyche and life.

- The three Magi who enter into the manger to worship the Christ-child are contrasted with the shepherds who remain outside, who recognize this great Event but who do not understand it. These archetypes thus represent two different and opposed types of human beings: the Magi represent the Faustian type who must go through the entire range of human experience and knowledge to finally arrive at the supreme Truth . . . if they do not stop on the way! The shepherds, on the other hand, represent the intuitive or mystical type who is drawn by the Truth and the Supreme Reality, without having to go through all the experiences and studies of the Faustian type.

- Gold, Myrrh and Frankincense, in the macrocosm, show symbolically how Jesus was recognized as a *King:* a being who is the master of himself and thus who can become a "channel" for the divine Will; as a *Priest*: a being who can act as transformer and projector for the Light, the spiritual energies, in this world; and as a *Prophet*: an initiate who can transmit and reveal the Mysteries.

- The fact that Mary could not find a place in the local inns and that Jesus had to be born in a manger tells us, symbolically, that the astral body and the consciousness of human beings are still so full of worldly desires and preoccupations that there is no "place" left for the spiritual energies and the divine Light . . . which must then wait before descending and dwelling in our heart.

- The Manger represents the psychospiritual center of the heart which is the "prism" through which the spiritual energies and the Light must "flow" so as to connect the conscious with the superconscious and the human with the spiritual Self. The presence in the Manger of the animals shows two essential things: first that the human heart still has "animal passions" when spiritual consciousness will be born and that these "animal passions", or biopsychic energies, must not be "repressed" or "killed" but rather "put to work" for the divine spark so that they can accomplish their "work" and "functions" in the biopsychic economy of human nature.

- Amongst the animals that are present at the birth of the Savior, the most important are the *bull* and the donkey which are basic archetypes. The bull represents the sexual energies while the *donkey* symbolizes the imagination and the stubbornness of the human ego. As these two are present and are breathing upon the Christ-child, they tell us in the symbolic language of the sacred traditions that sexual energies, the imagination and the determination of our personality must be integrated and put to work by the Light so that they can be transmuted and fulfill their natural functions and thus enable a human being to functionally become a child of God and a citizen of the Kingdom of Heaven.

- The star of the Savior, the Pentagram or five-pointed star, which guided the Magi to the Manger in Bethlehem, is the symbol of the *perfected soul* which descends from the spiritual worlds to incarnate on earth. This star is not visible on the physical plane but on the inner planes and requires a certain degree of clairvoyance to be seen. What this image tells us is that a Great Soul is coming to earth with an important and special mission. In the inner planes, each human being is literally a "star" and manifests his rank and spiritual level by his *light*. This is the same star that we will also find on top of the Christmas tree . . . which, again, is the symbol and the expression of a perfected human being, something we will all become some day.

- The Angels that sing "Glory to God in the highest and peace on earth to men of good will" represent the spiritual energies that flow between the human and the spiritual Self, between the field of consciousness and the superconscious. These have a profound impact upon our intuitions, thoughts, feelings and decisions. These psychospiritual energies will "light up" and "activate" the most important psychospiritual centers of our Tree of Life, bringing peace, harmony, and integration to the personality. "Glory" here simply refers to the spiritual light and splendor which always shines "above" and which are now recognized and experienced by the faithful. "Peace to men of good will" represents and establishes the true harmony between the psyche and its different levels, components and faculties which can now form a "living psychosynthesis"!

- The Christmas tree represents the Tree of Life, our psychospiritual centers and their paths, which we all have in our inner anatomy and physiology and which we must activate and "light up" for the inner Christ to be born in our psyche and to descend in our Tree of Life wherein He will dwell henceforth. Thus when we put a Christmas tree in our house, when we decorate it, light up its candles, and put a star on top, we are really projecting and *external symbol* of what we must realize and become internally: purify and sanctify our soul (decorate the tree), activate and illuminate its psychospiritual centers, and finally *become that tree* with its star on top (the symbol of a realized and perfected human being). When the divine will truly be born, will have awakened our spiritual consciousness, and will dwell in us consciously, this is exactly what will take place. In the inner worlds, we will literally appear as a "lit Christmas Tree" and be recognized as such by the spiritual powers and by those who possess the inner vision.

- During the Christmas holidays, human beings go to meet other human beings bringing cards and gifts to celebrate this Event and rejoice. All of this is a manifestation, on the physical plane, of what takes places on the inner planes at that moment. There is a great infusion of Light and spiritual energy which are poured into the atmosphere of the earth and into the aura of the person who lives his/her "personal Christmas". For then, the Spirit will give spiritual things: his Light, Life, and Being and human beings will respond in kind giving things that have meaning for them at their level of consciousness and being. Thus, when the divine is born and awakens in the human soul, in our being, it always brings many "gifts" together with the spirit of giving—a process which human beings recreate on their own levels.

- A final image and archetype related to the Christmas story is that of Santa Claus or St. Nicholas. Here we have an old man with white hair and a white beard, white gloves, who wears a red coat, travels with a flying reindeer around the world to bring presents to children. Who and what is this strange figure and archetype which is a composite of many symbols? It is none other than *ourselves*, not what we are today but what we can and will become tomorrow when we will be an "older soul". This is the reason why it has such a powerful appeal for our unconscious. An older soul has acquired wisdom (the white hair and beard), purity of heart (the white gloves), and can manifest spirit in matter (the red coat). It can also have out-of-the body experiences projecting his astral body and consciousness into the whole world. It looks upon human beings and the crazy things they do as "children who are playing (dangerous) games" . . . which are the best and most effective antidote for human folly and stupidity. Finally, it takes more pleasure in giving things (altruism) than in receiving them (egoism). Someday, we shall all become St. Claus and become like him and thus, unconsciously we can identify with him and take pleasure in his doings and adventures.

In conclusion, Christmas is truly the "image" or "blue-print" and the prototype and archetype of our own spiritual initiation—of the birth of God and of spiritual consciousness in our own souls . . . just as the Manger is the symbol and archetype of our own human heart (of the psychospiritual center of the heart and not the physical muscle, obviously!). It is the great Event towards which we are all moving, consciously and unconsciously, and which is prefigured and lived historically by the myth of the birth of Jesus and the archetype of the Manger . . . which are true and which will be realized someday by each and every human being.

It is also the central goal or objective of the Great Work of human growth and spiritual regeneration towards which all authentic psychological, human, and spiritual systems converge. Each one of these symbols, images, and archetypes, as well as the whole myth, can be used for doing much personal, psychological and spiritual work. Each one, of all of them, can be used as a theme and object for concentration, meditation, contemplation and theurgic work that integrate the functions of willing, thinking, feeling, imagination, and intuition to become actually what we are potentially and to fulfill our destiny on earth.

It is with in this spirit and with this wish that they are offered to you by tradition, in general, and in this work in particular. Specifically, each symbol and archetype can be used as a subject of meditation to decipher its deeper meanings and correspondences. For this is the only way in which we can make them "come alive" for us, in our consciousness, being, and life—by incarnating and incorporating them in our lives until such time as we shall reach and LIVE our own personal Christmas, or spiritual initiation. For, after all, this is the true reason for coming to earth and for undergoing all of the experiences and tests in the world of matter!

Chapter IV

THE EASTER STORY,
THE ARCHETYPE OF RESURRECTION

Easter is the greatest Christian celebration which takes place in the Spring. Buried in its symbols and images, the Easter archetype contains theoretical implications and practical applications that go way beyond its religious celebration and which apply to all human beings of all races, religions, and levels of consciousness. All the basic axioms and insights, together with the practical model we developed for the Christmas Story, also apply to and can be used with the Easter celebration and be extended to other celebrations, archetypes, symbols as well . . . as they can to other religions. The universality of the Easter Story as an anthropological and cosmic phenomenon can be seen very clearly given the fact that all religions have an important "holy day" and celebration at that time.

Thus, primitive cultures had the rites of Spring, the esoteric traditions the Spring Equinox, the Jews Passover, and the Muslim the great fast of Ramadan. This insight is further corroborated by the fact that when we carry out certain exercises and consciously cooperate with nature we, too, can experience certain results, live them in our consciousness and being and reap their benefits. The crucial period for this "experiment" begins mid-March and ends at the end of April; specifically it begins the 21st of March with the Spring Equinox and ends about seven weeks later. Lastly, if the message of Easter is not only religious but also anthropological and spiritual, then it must apply to *all human beings* regardless of their religion . . . or lack thereof.

By taking the spiritual tradition, the great primordial tradition, as our point of reference and perspective, we shall see that Easter, the Spring celebration, contains many meanings, implications and applications that can be very useful for human beings and for the world. Thus, the *Leitmotiv* of Easter on all planes of being is **rebirth** while for man, on the spiritual level it is **resurrection,** in that the resurrection of Jesus the Christ is truly an archetype for the resurrection of all human beings.

For nature, in the Spring, rebirth implies, as we can readily observe it, an awakening and rebirth of the whole of nature; it means that a new "life-wave" will now flow through the earth: the grass, the trees, the flowers, and the animal kingdom. Thus grass grows, the trees come alive and put on leaves and burgeons, flowers bloom and animals and birds wake from hibernation, and males chase females—the whole of nature comes alive and begins a new year as Life pours into its internal and external manifestations. The psychic and spiritual atmosphere of the world as well as the aura of human beings are "filled" and "bathe" in a new wave of life and energy that vivifies whatever it comes into contact with.

For Man, the same process of rebirth can manifest itself on four basic levels: the physical-vital, the emotional-astral, the mental and the spiritual level . . . but with one basic difference—human beings must *consciously participate* in this process while in nature it occurs naturally and *unconsciously* without the participation of those involved! Thus we must deliberately use all of our attention (will), thoughts (thinking), emotions (feeling) and visualization (imagination) if we want to obtain the best results. This because, having reached the present developmental stage, human evolution is now a *conscious process* which requires our full commitment and participation; whereas in nature evolution is still unconscious, responding to outer stimuli rather than to inner promptings.

It is also very important to remember what we pointed out in the previous chapter, namely that all symbols, archetypes, and religious celebrations contain not one but many meanings: implications and applications, which are a function of our level of consciousness and being as well as of our existential situation. As I have already pointed out several times before (but it bears repeating as this is a truly vital point), symbols, images, archetypes and myths can *veil* as well as *unveil*, hide or reveal certain truths, principles or laws depending on the level of consciousness and being as well as the discernment of the person who beholds and utilizes them.

The Easter myth can be fruitfully applied to two very different levels of our being: that of our *personality* (composed of the physical body, the etheric, astral, and mental bodies) which determine our awareness and behavior; and that of our *individuality* (or soul) which is made-up of our three higher energy bodies (the higher mental and the two spiritual ones). These together make up what we could call our lower and higher self. Let us begin by looking at and analyzing the meanings, implications and applications of Easter for our personality. Here there are three basic things that we can do, on three basic levels, to experience a cleansing and a revitalization—a literal rebirth—of our personality on its basic levels and which will last for about 6-9 months after which these will have to be repeated the following year

1. *Physical rebirth* (which we can consciously bring about during this period of the year) requires that a person directs all of her attention and efforts to bring about an internal and external house-cleaning. This implies purifying, equilibrating, and revitalizing one's physical body as well as coordinating recharging it with new energy and vitality. The Primordial Tradition has always taught that this can be accomplished by doing three things during this period of the year for at least for three consecutive weeks, namely beginning with a physical fast:

   - *Change your daily diet* (switching from meat and pasta to vegetables and fruits).
   - *Exposing your body to the elements (air and sunshine) and doing more physical exercise* (sports, yoga, breathing or calisthenics).
   - *Getting a little more sleep* (one to two more hours in the morning, evening or taking a siesta).

2. *Emotional rebirth* implies the purification, elevation, and intensification of our capacity to feel emotionally and to awaken new feelings and emotions. Beginning with an emotional fast (getting our emotions and feelings centered and avoiding strong negative or positive emotions), we can proceed with the following:

   - *Seeking beauty and becoming artistically involved* (with nature, with painting or music). Here, we must seek out and behold what we consider to be beautiful and harmonious. This because beauty, on all levels, is truly a nourishment for our psyche.
   - *Seeking out and interacting with people with whom we have affinities.* This means revitalizing our social life through conferences, travel, and visits. It could also be the appropriate time to make new acquaintances as well as nourishing and feeding existing ones.
   - *Using prayer in a regular fashion.* Here we can use silence and theurgy (concentration, meditation, devotion, and visualization resulting in a living invocation-evocation) to vivify our heart center and intensify our feelings and emotions.

3. *Mental rebirth* means the purification and expansion of our way of looking at and apprehending cognitively the world and our experiences in the world. It implies cleansing and dynamizing our ideas and our way of explaining what we are living through in the world and in ourselves.

Again, beginning with a mental fast (seeking to still our mind and empty it of all thoughts and ideas), there are three basic things we can do:

- *Reflecting, meditating and reading and writing on worthwhile topics.* This implies giving our mind good "food" by avoiding negative or trivial thoughts.
- *By seeking out and engaging in good conversations* with people who are on our wave-length and who can enrich us culturally and spiritually.
- *Through prayer and spiritual exercises* where the spiritual Light is now directed to our head psychospiritual center to activate it and vivify it.

The Christian celebration of Easter, however, is focused primarily upon the spiritual dimension where rebirth becomes a true *resurrection*. Symbolically and archetypally, this is represented by the Resurrection of Jesus on the third day. Resurrection here implies two basic things: First and foremost the awakening of the Christ within ourselves, of our divine spark which can then leave the "tomb" of our superconscious where it "sleeps" and awake at the conscious level in our heart center. Second, it also implies the development and crystallization of new *attitudes*, or ways of perceiving and responding to our lives and its tests and tribulations on higher levels of consciousness.

In particular, this involves the way in which we perceive and define ourselves, other human beings, good and evil, and the reason why we incarnated in this world. Essentially, this means to realize that Life has no beginning and no end, that we are spiritual and immortal beings; that both good and evil are serving God's ultimate Purpose and Plan hence, that they are both useful and have important functions to fulfill; and thus that all human experiences are, ultimately, a gift from God, and that as such they have a role to play in our becoming.

Spiritual resurrection can only come from the awakening and manifestation of *spiritual consciousness* which is the result of a true *spiritual initiation*. This spiritual initiation, in turn, is the result of perceiving and living Life as a "laboratory of personal growth" to develop one's character and integrity—one's soul; it is the result of praying in a conscious and living way and of coping with the great tests and trials of life with courage and personal integrity. This spiritual resurrection depends, more than upon psychospiritual exercises, knowledge and techniques, upon our *level of consciousness* and *being*, upon our purity and holiness which are grounded in what *we are* rather than upon what *we do*!

The central axis of this resurrection is that of the *love of God* and of the *love of our fellow human beings* where an important key is *fasting* and *praying*, generosity and altruism. The love of God is manifested by drawing closer to Him (in terms of our consciousness, energies and vibrations) by filling our energy bodies and their psychospiritual centers with His Light, Fire, and Life, and by harmonizing our consciousness and will with His. The love of our fellow human beings is expressed through genuine *service* which consists not in satisfying the demands and caprices of the other, but by helping him grow and achieving true autonomy and personal integrity.

Fasting here involves not only the physical dimension (abstaining from eating or eating less) but also to deprive our energy bodies of their usual nourishment: controlling or eliminating certain emotions, desires, thoughts, conversations, and states of being. It consists in *emptying* ourselves if we wish to put something else in our consciousness and being! Prayer, which is the complementary polarity of fasting, consists in *filling* ourselves to replace the void created by fasting with better things: more light, wisdom, warmth, love, life and creative energies.

Fasting on the three basic levels of the personality (physical-vital, emotional-astral and mental) corresponds to the phase of *purification*; whereas prayer corresponds, on the same three levels, to the phase of *consecration*. And it is precisely during this period of the year that we can make, with our brothers and sisters, "conscious efforts" and accept "voluntary sufferings" which are the substance of a true sacrifice (from the Latin: *sacrum facere*, to make holy and not to deprive ourselves of something). This entails a true "alchemy", or exchange, whereby we replace something "below" with something "above". For example, replacing physical gold (material wealth) with spiritual gold (the ability to know, to love, and to create) or physical love (which is essentially egoistical) with spiritual love (which is essentially altruistic).

Spiritual resurrection, or spiritual rebirth, requires not only a new and higher state of consciousness and being, but also a new and higher perception and comprehension of the meaning and purpose of Life and of its trials and tribulations on earth. Thus, this resurrection touches and affects all of our psychospiritual centers and chakras engendering new attitudes and responses to the challenges that daily life brings to each and every one of us. Specifically:

1. At the level of the *first chakra*: this involves the struggle for *physical survival* with all of its fears, anxieties, anger and frustrations which are now transformed into an authentic *acceptance and gratitude* for all those things that we can be called to experience and live through and for facing the tests and tribulations that are now before us. Those whose vital energies are blocked at the level of the first chakra will, inevitably, develop a hypertrophy of this center which creates an "existential anxiety" or anguish and a compulsive fear of being unable to survive at the biological level. This, in turn, will generate as a reaction a violent desire and an aggressiveness to obtain as much money as possible that

should ensure their physical survival. But this, in turn, will create all sorts of dysfunctional attitudes and behaviors (e.g. the fear of biological death, greed, avarice, egoism, and conflicts of all sorts). To move through this particular phase is one of the great trials of life on earth which is represented, archetypally, by the first temptation of Jesus in the desert.

2.   At the level of the *second chakra*: this involves the struggle for *emotional survival* which depends upon our ability to have or to find a romantic/ sexual partner. The primordial fear here is that of "dying emotionally" if nobody loves us; it is the existential anxiety of solitude and of having to "live alone". These must now be transformed into true *courage*, the courage to be and to live "alone" if necessary and *integrity*, remaining true to our self. Thus, it implies moving beyond the fear of not being loved at the romantic and sexual level—to have at least one person who perceives us and feels that we are unique and indispensable for our well-being. Those whose vital energies are blocked at the level of the second chakra will also develop a hypertrophy of this center which creates an "existential anxiety" or anguish and a compulsive fear of not being able to survive at the emotional level. This, in turn, will generate a violent desire and a compulsion to always have someone who is "in love with us". But this will also create various dysfunctional attitudes and behaviors (e.g. love as a game or conquest, the complex of the play-boy or *femme fatale*, and the search for superficial relationships which are constantly replaced by other such relationships). To move beyond this phase is another of the great trials of life which is represented, archetypally by the second temptation of Jesus in the desert.

3.   At the level of the *third chakra*: this implies the struggle for power, the need to feel "important" and "admired" by others—the compulsion to be materially and socially successful. This will now be transformed in true *contentment* with what one is and what one has; with the living faith that we already *have everything* that is truly important and essential for our wellbeing at this time. Those whose vital energies are blocked at the level of the third chakra will, inevitably, develop a hypertrophy of this center that will then create an "existential anxiety" and a compulsive fear of not being able to survive at the social, professional, and intellectual level. The reaction engendered by this will be a violent desire, an obsession for being truly "special and important" for others—a true addiction to the power complex. This will then produce various kinds of dysfunctional attitudes and behaviors (e.g. becoming a workaholic, exploiting and manipulating others as "things", repressing one's feelings, and losing one's inner harmony and balance). Moving beyond this phase is yet another great test of life which corresponds, archetypally, to the third temptation of Jesus in the desert.

4. At the level of the *fourth chakra*: we find the great "passage" or "turning-point" going from the personality to the soul, from our lower to our higher nature. It is here that we find the "death of the personality" and the "resurrection of the individuality"—the birth of spiritual consciousness in our soul. Through this process, we become aware of our soul and we want to make Christ become our Lord (i.e. the unifying and integrating principle of our psyche and behavior). This center can be subdivided, just as is the physical heart (!) into two basic parts: the lower and the higher part. The lower part engenders "soft love" (doing everything that the other wants so that he/she will not suffer and will not reject us); whereas the higher part engenders "tough love (doing what is truly best for the growth and well being of the other) which requires wisdom, self-knowledge and self-mastery. Here, the need for social approval and the inability to say "no" to others who demand all kinds of things from us cease. Thus it is here that we will cease to "sell our own conscience and integrity for the need to be loved and accepted". These will now be transmuted into genuine *compassion*—the ability to see and to feel through the eyes and the heart of the other without losing or betraying one's self. In a nutshell, this is the great test of love—wise or foolish love as Dante would say!

5. At the level of the *fifth chakra*: we develop the need and aspiration to discover the *essential principles of Life* and to understand the *law of cause and effect* in the world and in ourselves. This leads us by degrees to develop an authentic and personal sense of responsibility—to understand and live in accordance with the great laws of God and Life.

6. At the level of the *sixth chakra*: we develop the need and aspiration to learn how to *love unconditionally*—to accept the other exactly as he/she is with all his/her strengths and weaknesses. Thus we now develop the capacity to experience reality as does the other—to enter into his own consciousness and view-point. And this will bring us to an unconditional acceptance of the other and to truly put ourselves in his service so as to live and become SPIRITUAL LOVE!

7. Finally, at the level of the *seventh chakra*: we acquire the need and the capacity to *let God express Himself within our own consciousness and life*. This, in turn, will engender and manifest itself as authentic *humility*. This means not being afraid of living "the ordinary life of an ordinary person" but bringing through and expressing divine Light, Fire and Life or the wisdom, love and creative energies of God in our being and in our daily life.

Once a person has truly lived and experienced his personal resurrection at the spiritual level, he will truly develop a "new consciousness" and a "new being" that will enable him to now face and accept all the aspects and dimensions of himself and all the trials and tribulations of Life without *fear* and without *guilt*—without rejecting or repressing anything whatever! And it is only at this point that that person can live the old Roman saying "nihil humanum alienum a me puto" (that is, nothing that is human will be alien to me; I will not reject or be afraid of anything that Life can throw at me!).

Unfortunately most people, most of the time, are blocked, limited and driven by their fears and anxieties, by their personal traumas and desires. Thus, they are not yet able—so long as they are only functioning at their personality level—to experience the greatest miracle and the most important human accomplishment which consists in being able to *live life fully and consciously, without fear and without guilt.* And this is what spiritual resurrection truly makes possible for all those who live through it and have experienced it. To conclude, let me cite what I wrote at the end of 1986 in a book that was called "Apocalypse Now" by my publisher (Llewellyn, 1988):

"It is at this point, when Resurrection, our "personal Easter", really occurs that we finally know who we are, where we come from, where we are going, and what we have come on earth to accomplish; that we shall find and be able to use the Philosopher's Stone, the Elixir Vitae, and the Panacea; that our higher Self, the Lord, can truly "come unto His Kingdom" and "inhabit His temple"; and that the mystery and paradox of good and evil can finally be understood and resolved . . . and that Man will, once again, become the potential God he is and, thereby, reacquire his immortality, bliss, and sinlessness. No more can be usefully said at this point about this great event . . . which must be *personally lived and experienced* to be truly understood and realized".

Chapter V

GRACE AND SPIRITUAL ENERGY

In the present chapter, we are going to look at three basic concepts and insights which, together, will enable us to gain greater closure on the fascinating and most important concept of grace and spiritual energy: the nature, dynamics and expressions of grace and spiritual energy, their relationship to human effort, and the two realms of Nature and Grace. Together, these insights will help us to better understand, appreciate, and utilize the emerging laws, principles, and energies that are making "miracles" possible and which will enable us to cope with the tremendous challenges of our times—to avoid its dangers and to profit from its opportunities. Even more important, they will enable us to live through and do our part in the great passage and transformation of our consciousness and being that will lead to from childhood into true adulthood through the "crisis of adolescence" and its final "maturity exam".

One of the greatest mysteries and gifts is unquestionably that of *Life*! With Life everything is possible without it nothing is possible, neither the greatest evil nor the highest good! But what is Life? Life is life-force, vitality or energy. What is energy, where does it come from, what are its deeper nature, dynamics, purpose, and manifold manifestations? These are very profound questions that thinkers in many disciplines have wondered upon and sought to answer for as long as human beings have lived on earth and have been able to think, ask questions, and express their curiosity.

One of the deepest intuitions and insights of the Sages and Seers of antiquity and now also one of the latest and most promising discoveries and realizations of the modern science are all converging towards the same basic conclusion: the Universe, Life, and Reality are composed of energies and vibrations with an *infinity of quantitative and qualitative frequencies*. So Life and Reality really come from the same Source and are, ultimately, the same thing . . . even though

Life does not come from matter but "inhabits" it or manifests through it, as it were. Life comes from *elsewhere*, from the Spirit, and expresses itself through matter. Life is energy, an energy that is clearly *multidimensional* with three basic expressions which are physical, psychic, and spiritual energy.

From a scientific viewpoint, energy is a force that brings about transformations, basic changes, which are empirically observable, and the actualization of potentialities. For example, movement, growth, development and consciousness are all measurable consequences of some form of energy. Vibrations are measurable in terms of their frequencies and amplitudes that manifest themselves in a sinusoidal form and as "spirals" that can be ascending or descending (i.e. increasing their level of organization and vitality or decreasing them). Energy is thus an expression of Life, of the cosmic force which, like all aspects of creation, can find expression on three great qualitative planes or aspects: the physical, the human or psychic, and the spiritual.

On the physical plane, energy is the force, of the manifestation of Life, which brings about an observable change (movements in space, transformations of weight and volume, a change in temperature, and growth or decay). On the human level, energy is the force that nourishes, transforms, and actualizes our potentialities, the most important of which is *consciousness*. Finally, on the spiritual plane, energy comes from Life which is its source and essence, and which animates or ensouls matter, evolution, and the creation and expression of self. Spiritual energy is thus primordial Life without which there could be no creation, evolution of manifestation of any kind.

In human nature, energy manifests itself upon four qualitatively different planes, that is:

1. On the physical level as a vital force capable of moving, growing, and utilizing matter to act and grow on the space-time continuum.
2. On the emotional level, as an emotive force capable of feeling, reacting emotionally, and as courage or the desire to live, with passion and appreciation . . . or their opposites, through the wide range of experiences that Life can bring.
3. On the mental plane as a rational-cognitive force, or capacity to understand and organize coherently one's experience in the world and within one's own psyche.
4. On the spiritual plane, as love-force relating and binding one's self, others, God, and Life itself. Here energy is *faith* which brings us to open ourselves to Life and its multiples experiences, adventures, tests, and trials.

At the phenomenological level, spiritual energy manifests itself as Light, Fire, and Life; that is, as the fundamental impulsion behind human consciousness and everything that vivifies and animates it. Structurally speaking, when spiritual energy flows through or manifests within the Tree of Life (our psychospiritual centers according to the Western spiritual tradition), it manifests as Light or Wisdom; when it flows through the head psychospiritual center which implies consciousness and knowledge as Fire or Love, when it flows through the heart psychospiritual center and implies desire and sensibility. And as Creative energy or Will, when it flows through our shoulder psychospiritual centers and implies the ability to create and express one's self.

At the functional level, an intellectual will perceive spiritual energy as Light or understanding; an artist or emotional person as Fire or passion and sensibility; and an active, physical type of person, as a vital force or current. Finally, a mystic, a spiritually awakened person, will perceive spiritual energy as Life-force with its three empirical manifestations as Light, Fire, and Life—the life-giving and vivifying energy that activates and nourishes his intuition and his entire consciousness with its manifold manifestations. This Life-force will then bring about the unfoldment of "self-consciousness", will reconnect that person with his Source and vivify or "light up" all the psychospiritual centers on his Tree of Life and make all the functions of his psyche "come alive" and able to express themselves.

Spiritual energy is known and called by different names in different traditions and in its multiple manifestations. For example, it has been called "grace", the "power of the Holy Spirit", "spiritual gold", "prana", "chi" or "cosmic energy". Of all the things that human beings covet and have been seeking, spiritual energy or grace, is by far the most important, what is "essential par excellence", because without it there can be no life, love, consciousness, self-expression or anything! It is literally, in its multiple expressions, the "essence or fuel" of life, of consciousness, of love, and of self-expression which cannot exist without it.

In other words, without spiritual energy, there cannot be life, consciousness, love, sensibility, motivation, health, creativity or joy! It is therefore the "gift of God" par excellence, the most important and precious thing there is which, by bringing life and its life-giving force, gives existence and value to everything else. Like and immense river, it comes from the "heart of God", of our divine spark, to flow through and manifest in the seven great planes of creation and human nature in order to "activate, nourish, and develop" human consciousness . . . and thus enabling man to consciously return to his Source.

Today, we are living at a most interesting and unusual historical juncture and point of our human evolution which is characterized by great paradoxes, contradictions, seeming injustices, and confusion. Our epoch has been called and characterized in different ways by different traditions. The Judeo-Christian tradition calls it the "Apocalypse" (not the end of the world but the "revelation of a hidden truth" or the "opening of the unconscious and superconscious" according to its etymological meaning), the Easter tradition calls it the "Kali Yuga", the Amerindians the "Period of the Great Purification or Tribulation", the classical Greco-Roman tradition, the "Iron Age", whereas I like to call it the "crisis of adolescence" culminating in the "maturity exam" which we will all have to live through within a few years.

In a nutshell, this is the period in which we are going through a very major expansion and transformation of consciousness, moving from "childhood" to "adulthood", wherein very great and real dangers and horrors exist but also even greater opportunities and marvels. This is the time wherein Life, Evolution, or the higher Powers are in fact saying to us: "move to a higher level of consciousness and being or perish at your own hands"! Focusing on the tremendous paradoxes, contradictions and confusion of our times we find:

- The "project Man", as conceived by the great Power and Intelligence that created us, was to unfold gradually and bring about the God-Man; but it seems that we have (at least temporarily) replaced this by the cancer-man!
- For more than two centuries, we have been told that, through reason, science, and proper education and discipline, we would bring about great and ongoing *progress*. Thus, life on earth should become easier, more comfortable and predictable, yet everyday reality reveals that we have brought about its opposite: life is becoming evermore complex, complicated and difficult so that more and more people, in more and more places, are now becoming unable to cope with the growing demands and challenges of life.
- It is true that at the material and external level, human beings have never had so much: so much knowledge, education, social and political freedom, money, and technology, and yet . . . human beings have never been so confused, miserable, and depressed at the human and inner level!

Not only, but the world is also becoming an ever-more violent place where outer and inner conflicts, social, economic, and political struggles as well as physical and psychological diseases are now proliferating and getting out of control. Hence, confusion, pessimism, and cynicism on the part of many people are growing . . . as are various addictions and "escapes from reality" such as alcohol, drugs (legal and illegal), sex, money, and power. For if reality no longer makes sense, if it is not worth our efforts and sacrifices, then we will want to "get away from it", deny it, destroy it, or put it behind us! So how can we explain these paradoxes and confusion? There are, of course, many different ways of look at and answering this complex and puzzling situation.

For me, however, one thing is becoming ever-more clear, as I travel in different countries and interact with various types of people: the black box of science, reason and our senses, and *human effort* are no longer enough if we arc to survive and live well in the 21st Century! We need something else, something qualitatively different which is *divine grace* (spiritual energies): higher laws, principles, and energies to meet the growing challenges of our times and the growing complexities of our society. What we need is to move from one basic level of consciousness to another—from the personality to the soul—and for that we need *grace*, a higher intelligence, energy, and inspiration that those of the human ego and of the personality. This is why the 21st Century will, indeed, be spiritual . . . or will not be!

Humanism: human efforts, the development of our ego and personality, the refinement of our thinking, feeling, and will processes, the cultivation of reason, the senses and our will can only lead us ultimately to materialism, reductionism, egoism, and hedonism; to want to pursue the temporal *good of the part* at the expenses of the long-range *good of the whole*. It leads us to wild scientific, social, political, and religious experimentation which will yet raise the level of confusion, conflict, and despair further . . . as we raise our level of knowledge, will and power. This because the more aggressive and interventionist we become with our human ego and personality, the more and the greater the number of problems that we will create.

Both human nature and the nature of the universe and of Life are far more complex and multidimensional that we ever thought or can imagine! This, in turn, means that there are great imponderables and unknowns pertaining to the consequences and the "ripple-effect" we set in motion when we intervene and change something in the part . . . that ends up by affecting the whole! This, I believe, is where we are today and what characterizes our present historical juncture. What we need, to begin with, is a *proper perspective* or theoretical framework to enable us to better understand what we truly are, why we incarnated in this world, what kind of a world and historical period we are presently living in, and what we can do to get "back on the tracks" of our destiny and purpose.

To do this, to promote the "good of the whole", to achieve true peace, health, morality, fulfillment and joy, we need higher inspiration, guidance, energies and faculties—we need *divine grace*! We need to be able to consciously access the Light, which is also Love and Life, the Source that created both the universe and ourselves and which, obviously, knew what it was doing! We need to go back to what is truly *essential* which, by definition, is what is simple, natural, moral, non-dangerous, and inexpensive! We need an appropriate "frame of reference" and "yard-stick" which, obviously, cannot be the average person, certainly not the pathological person and not even the successful secular person. We need Saints, Sages, and Prophets, people who have reached higher levels of consciousness and being, who have activated their intuition and awakened their spiritual consciousness!

So what is divine grace? It is quite complex and, ultimately, an ineffable mystery, treasure, and free gift that must be *experienced and lived personally* to be properly understood! Any intellectual definition of it and attempt to gain cognitive closure of its nature, dynamics and possibilities can only remain partial and inadequate and yet it is what I will attempt to do to provide you with a "blue-print" of some of them so as to motivate you to the personal work necessary to receive it and experience it. Grace involves the set of higher energies, laws, and frequencies that can reach us at the *interdimensional* level by coming down the planes and our levels of consciousness as it were. Through human effort we can purify, consecrate, and coordinate our Tree of Life and its psychospiritual centers, our aura or "energy bodies", our consciousness and personality, and our endocrine and nervous system to be receptive to them, to invite them, and to become a good "temple" or "instrument" for them to manifest through us.

While human effort is the "work of the moon", divine grace is the "work of the sun" which can be graphically represented by a downward pointing triangle so that, having done our part through human effort, we can now ask for help both at the horizontal level (from other human beings) and at the vertical level (from God). Grace thus complements and completes what we have begun with human effort (represented by an upward pointing triangle) and represents the connection and union of spirit and matter, of God and man, which can be graphically represented by the Star of David.

At the spiritual level, grace is the Uncreated Light which can manifest and prismate itself into Light, Fire, and Life and which consists of an infinite range of energies and frequencies, the very "stuff" the universe and reality are made of and which modern science is just now beginning to discover, study, and integrate. This Light or energy is everywhere but originates and dwells in higher dimensions than our own. Through various "transformers, condensers and projectors" and, ultimately, through *human beings*, it can manifest downwards so as to eventually reach the physical level to mold it and fashion it into its own original plan and model—into the Kingdom of Heaven.

Grace is everywhere but must be "invited" in order to flow into us and manifest consciously through our being and it will do so, gradually and progressively, as we get ready for it and desire it. A good analogy here would be that of an electrical machine that can operate on a certain electrical voltage (say 120 volts). If we raise that voltage, speed and frequencies so as to improve its performance and capabilities (say to 10,000 volts), it is clear that we have to work upon it and adapt it to higher levels. Exactly the same thing happens with our personality and grace: we must prepare and condition our personality (our Tree of Life and its psychospiritual centers as well as our hormonal and nervous system) otherwise we would burn ourselves and fry our circuits!

Perhaps a simple but extreme example of that would be self-combustion whereby people burn themselves and their immediate environment by developing extremely high temperatures and heat (which, psychically, would imply activating certain psychospiritual centers prematurely and when we cannot yet handle their energies and frequencies). Thus, there is a long and organic "preparation" for the reception and utilization of grace which the mystics call: purification, consecration and union with God.

The theoretical implications and the practical applications of grace and spiritual energy are enormous and, as yet, unfathomable. They will be revealed to us progressively as they come, dwell in, and manifest through us. In a nutshell, grace can inspire us and guide us (activate our intuition) so that we know exactly what is "good" and what is "bad" for us, what is the "right dose" and the "proper moment" for something . . . which our reason cannot provide as it would take an infinitely long period of time to obtain the precise and optimal information. Grace and higher spiritual energies can, likewise, heal us of all of our infirmities and dysfunctions by re-establishing and re-creating the proper *bio-psycho-spiritual harmony* and by supplying the necessary energy and materials. Grace can also bestow upon us a sense of joy, fulfillment, and ecstasy that is truly indescribable and which, again, must be personally experienced to be properly known and understood.

Grace can help us solve the enigma of the Sphinx and reveal to us who we are, whence we come, wither we are going, what we have come to do in this world, and what we are meant to become. Thus, it can reveal to us the mystery and paradox of God, or Reality, of Life; of the universe, of good and evil, of joy and suffering as well as their deeper meanings, implications and applications in our lives and in our evolution. Grace especially implies having a *life more abundant*, through understanding the deeper meaning of life, and being able to live it, appreciate it, and be grateful for it in rising degrees of intensity and awareness. It is also grace that will enable us to move from living in an unconscious to an ever-more conscious way; that is, in a responsible, autonomous, productive, healthy, moral, creative and joyful way!

In conclusion, grace and spiritual energies complete and complement human efforts and physical and psychic energies through a feed-back loop where each activates and intensifies, or harmonizes the other, thus helping us to complete our being, actualize our faculties and potentialities, and fulfill our destiny: to become what we were meant to be! It is the authentic Saints, Sages, Prophets and Mystics (those who have achieved higher levels of consciousness and being) who have shown, spoken about and demonstrated the existence of grace and some of its wondrous potentialities and possibilities. And it is Jesus the Christ, the realized God-Man, and the Prototype and Archetype for all human beings, Who incarnated, lived, and demonstrated, in the fullest fashion possible, that grace exists, that we can receive it, and some of the things that it can mean and do for us.

On a lower level, when I was a child and for a certain period of time, I had access to the inner worlds and could see some things that most people do not see, including some of manifestations of grace or Light. For example, when going to Mass and participating in Communion, I would notice that the consecrated host would become "radioactive", that like a little sun it would radiate Light, Fire and Life, if you had the inner vision open to perceive this. This "radiation" however, took place in a rather strange and paradoxical way. It would radiate 360 degrees around like one would expect light and photons to radiate, touching everything within its radius. Yet, it would also "shoot some pointed rays" to one or two rare persons.

As for the "reception and assimilation" of this light and energy, I also witnessed something very particular, paradoxical, and fascinating: for most people, the Light, Fire, and Life the energies radiated by the consecrated Eucharist would simply flow *around their energy-bodies*, or aura, but they would not penetrate into them or they would penetrate to a very slight extent! The rare person would have one of the "special rays" directed towards himself/herself or who would receive the Eucharist may have this Light, Fire, and Life actually flow *right into their energy bodies* and would then light-up and activate one or more psychospiritual center. Their aura would then become much larger and more brilliant and they would literally "light-up" and even help "light-up" some of the people near them!

As time went by, I grew and matured and became more curious and intrigued by this paradoxical phenomenon. Thus I decided to talk to the two types of persons to see what kind of experience they had, to what extent these experienced differed, and what might be the implications of these differences. I discovered that the people for whom the Light, Fire, and Life flowed around their energy-bodies did not experience much of anything and certainly no changes or transformations. They felt good and stated they had done their "religious duty" by participating in an important rite but that practically nothing happened at a conscious level.

Those for whom these energies actually penetrated into their aura and Tree of Life stated that something very "real and powerful" had taken place but which they did not fully understand. They had felt "filled with light, life, and joy" and wanted to do great things; that "something" had touched them and vivified them! This taught me that grace, the uncreated Light and the spiritual energies, are received and integrated by people in a very different way, which was directly related to their level of consciousness and being, to their preparation and receptivity, and was not standardized or made uniform for all those who participated in it.

In conclusion, grace is spiritual energy, Light, that can come down through the planes or "interdimensionally", enter into and fill our being. Its major, overall impact is to vivify our entire being and to reconnect our psyche to our soul (our field of consciousness with our superconscious and our human with our spiritual Self) and to make our unconscious conscious! It generally "prismates" itself into Light (when flowing through the mind), Fire (when flowing through the heart) and Life or vital energies (when flowing through our shoulder centers). As Light, it raises and vivifies our consciousness, providing understanding and inspiration; as Fire, it activates and vivifies our love, providing taste, feeling, motivation, appreciation and desire; as Life, it dynamizes and vivifies our will and our creative energies enabling us to express ourselves, to act and to create.

Hence, it provides the "force" polarity which must be complemented and completed with the "form" polarity; in other words, life and energy must have an "instrument" and a "receptacle" through which they can manifest. For without such a "vehicle", the Light and Fire could not be "fixed" and would dissipate; whereas the "vehicle" without the Light and energy would remain lifeless, like a computer without electricity! In the spiritual life, human effort generally culminates in and is epitomized by "asceticism" whereas grace culminates and is epitomized by "mysticism". Clearly, both are very important and must be brought together and properly integrated. When they are, then they can lead to the transformation and slow maturation of the animal-man into the God-Man.

First, we need a *metanoia* or conversion, a change of heart that will lead us to change our values and priorities from the world and temporal things to God and eternal things. Then will come the three basic steps of *catharsis, fotisis,* and *theosis,* namely the systematic purification, consecration, illumination, and deification whereby we reach our ultimate end and fully realize our destiny. The interesting point here is that to continue and complete our evolution and reach perfection, namely our gradual transformation into the God-Man, we need both *human effort* and *divine grace,* but in varying degrees. We might begin with some balance between them, then pass on to a major focus and emphasis upon human effort (our present stage), but to eventually balance them again, and then gradually privilege grace . . . that will complete the Great Work!

A final angle or viewpoint from which we can look at the question of grace and spiritual energy is that of the two realms or fundamental laws: that of *nature* (on the horizontal dimension) and that of *grace* (on the vertical dimension). These two "realms" or basic "laws" can rationally explain one of the most interesting paradoxes of the Holy Scriptures: "What is impossible for men is possible for God"; in other words, many of the so-called "miracles" attributed to God still remain "arbitrary" and "unexplainable" or "unintelligible" for us. This can be simply put into perspective and rationally explained by saying that: as we move on from the "realm of nature" to that of "grace", and are thus able to draw upon, at the *interdimensional level,* higher energies and frequencies, we can do or witness, over a very short period of time, things that would truly be impossible at the level of the "realm of nature" and that would remain "opaque" or unexplainable at a rational level.

This distinction and insight are thus a truly essential key to unite science and spirituality and to provide a modern and rational explanation able to integrate opposites and thus reconcile faith and reason. After all, if God has endowed us with the faculties of reason and intelligence, it is so that we can develop and utilize them. Postulating the multidimensionality of reality, both internal and external, something that mathematics and science have now demonstrated, we are now able to render intelligible and to reconcile the opposed polarities of determinism and freedom, of law and compassion, and of the inner and outer aspects of reality. Science clearly begins "below" to slowly move "upwards" to explain the phenomena of nature, whereas spirituality begins "above" to slowly descend "below", working with intuition, inspiration, and spiritual vision to enable us to understand our being and our experiences.

Given these premises, it is clear that, at a certain level of consciousness and point of human evolution, these two approaches will meet . . . half way along this continuum. For me, this "period of time" is clearly today (circa 1950 to 2050). This is, indeed, the "time of horrors" but also the "time of wonders and miracles" when God, the Light, intervenes in a more conscious and intense way in our consciousness as well as in the world. Thus far an "abyss" has always separated empirical science from revealed religion. This "abyss" pitted against each other reason and logic vs. faith and emotional sensibility as it did the determinism of natural laws and the freedom of choice and expression. Today, if I am right, we will be able to dissolve this "abyss" and to unite and reconcile these opposites.

Personally, I have never believed in so-called "miracles" or arbitrary and incomprehensible manifestations of a capricious divinity that portrays, at a higher level, human nature. I believe, rather, that there are many higher energies, principles, and laws that we are yet very far from understanding or even able to imagine . . . which could explain extraordinary phenomena . . . a little bit like a primitive person would be unable to understand the nature and dynamics of a computer, a cell phone, or a television set that, for him, would appear as "magic". Amongst these "extraordinary phenomena", we find in particular the sensational, almost instantaneous, complete and lasting *healings* brought about by Saints, Sages, and authentic healers, even though they latter lacked all types of professional training or clinical experience, and who can succeed where conventional medicine is helpless.

In the above, we find a concrete and practical example of what I call the "Great Paradox of medicine" which has created major antagonism and contrasts between conventional healthcare practitioners and healers. This "Great Paradox" is the fact that there have always been men and women, of all races and religions, who, without professional training or clinical experience, were able to bring about exceptional complete, definitive and almost instantaneous healings in cases that were clearly and explicitly called incurable by conventional medicine. Some of the best known examples of these are Padre Pio, the Curé d'Ars, Maître Philippe de Lyons and Bruno Groening.

To take a very simple and yet profound image from Bruno Groening: a human being is like a battery that burns up energy. God is the central electrical power station and the Saints and Healers are the transformers, condensers, and projectors of spiritual energy. A person who is sick or suffering must open-up, become receptive and invite this Life or energy to come into her being, to live and vivify her being and consciousness and thus to re-establish proper *bio-psycho-spiritual harmony*. Here the focal point is no longer the physical body, which is studied by biochemistry and which is subdivided into anatomy and physiology; rather, it is the *energy-bodies* (specifically, the etheric, emotional mental, and spiritual body with their psychospiritual centers) that become the focus of attention and intervention.

The essential element here is Life, or energy (the *Vis Vitalis*). With the new buzz-word of "PNEI axis" (the old *Vis Medicatrix Naturae* or the immune, hormonal, nervous and circulatory systems), the new medicine of the energy-bodies and spiritual medicine in particular can now explain, in very simple and rational language, how these exceptional healings can occur. With the proper energy and frequencies, these systems of auto-repair and regeneration (activating the etheric matrix and the DNA) can do their work in a very short period of time. When we speak of "energy" and "frequencies" we are turning into and contacting the *vertical dimension*, the interdimensional axis of our being and consciousness. These give us the possibility to rise to the higher "floors" of the inner sky-scraper and thus to pass from the realm of Nature to that of Grace; or, in other words, to be able to access higher laws, principles and frequencies then the ones that we know and that already exist on higher levels, but in a state of latency.

Even though many of their characteristics are different and opposed, there exists a continuum between these two realms. The realm of Nature is the realm of matter, of physical energy with well-defined and precise laws and principles that are universal and ruled by an iron *determinism*: to given causes correspond given effects. In simple words, the realm of Nature is the realm of the world. The realm of Grace, on the other hand, is the realm of spirit and spiritual energy which is also ruled by very precise and well-defined laws and principles and whose distinctive characteristic is *freedom*. This is the realm of man and of the spirit.

To give a concrete example which I had already mentioned briefly, the realm of Nature is like a machine which operates with 120 volts whereas the realm of Grace is like a machine that can utilize up to 12,000 volts. The first will, obviously be more limited, both at the quantitative and at the qualitative level, than the second which could do things that are impossible for the first! Following this analogy, to raise the efficiency and performance of the given machine, we need to adjust its electrical circuits and rheostats for a higher voltage. In the case of human beings, it is our consciousness and being, our energy-bodies and their psychospiritual centers that must be adapted to the higher energies and frequencies.

To be able to receive and use these higher energies and frequencies, it is necessary to provide inner and outer "transformers" and "condensers" that are able to handle them. This means conditioning our hormonal and nervous systems, our energy bodies and their psychospiritual centers which, in turn, require a certain level of consciousness, a certain life-style and state of mind that are in harmony with the laws of life. In particular, it requires a certain awareness and consonance with the divine Will and Plan. For, without this, these higher energies and frequencies could create an enormous chaos and conflict in the world as well as in our being and lives! To give too much knowledge and power to people who would use them for personal and egoistical ends would entail risks and a catastrophe which were not foreseen by divine providence!

Up to our present historical period, with the exception of a few great souls (Saints, Sages, and spiritually awakened persons), we have remained under the rule of the personality and thus enclosed in the realm of Nature, of the external physical world and of its four elements. It is this realm, with its universal and deterministic laws, that science has dealt with up, to the present time, and this is one of the reasons why science stood in opposition to religion which, at least in its essence, has always looked upon and aimed at the realm of Grace.

Having reached the present stage and level of consciousness and being, when we are, collectively, moving from what I call the "person of talent" to the "disciple", or from the rule of the personality to that of the soul, we will, once again, be able to recognize and enter into the realm of Grace, integrating it in our consciousness, being and life. And by doing so, we will be able to access and benefit from the higher laws and principles that it entails. To a certain extent, this is what occurred, but in the opposite direction, with the famous "Fall" and "expulsion from the garden of Eden" of the Holy Scriptures. At that time we moved from the realm of Grace to that of Nature where we have been up to the present historical juncture.

This second passage, through our transformation and expansion of consciousness, will also enable religion to move from the "tribal" level to the universal one and will make it possible for us to bring about a synthesis of religion, science, philosophy, and literature, thus creating a "compendium of human knowledge" that will include all academic disciplines—the famous "encyclopedia" of the Age of Reason and the Philosopher Stone of the esoteric traditions.

The basic insight and process that can render intelligible and rational the nature, dynamics, and manifestations of the realm of Grace is that of the *interdimensionality* of both man and the cosmos; the fact that both (as man is the imagine and synthesis of the later) contain not only a *quantitative* (from the smallest to the biggest) but also a *qualitative* (from spirit to matter and vice versa) dimension. These can render intelligible and explain rationally the manifestations and consequences of the higher laws and energies in both human nature and in the world.

For Reality is such (both at the outer and at the inner levels) that it is made of an infinity of energies and frequencies that can *transform themselves* and express themselves both at the *horizontal* (quantitative and external) level and at the *vertical* (qualitative and internal) level. This brings about what has rightly been termed the "Great Chain of Being" which connects (and enables communication) between the whole of creation and its Creator . . . moving up and down the "Ladder of Jacob" which is made up of a multitude of qualitative dimensions that are connected and that can communicate with each other.

As the universe is in expansion, so are our consciousness and being. At the present historical juncture and with the level of consciousness and being that we have now reached, we are called to become *adults* and thus to pass from the realm of Nature to that of Grace, to unite grace to human effort, the female polarity to the male, the external, objective aspect of reality with its internal and subjective one, and matter with spirit. In other words, we are now called to *reconcile opposites* rather than pitting one against the other and forcing people to choose between the one or the other—we are called to add the realm of Grace to that of Nature and thus to integrate both science and religion in a *living spirituality*. By so doing, we will be able to activate our intuition and awaken our spiritual consciousness . . . which will make it possible for us to rediscover and enter into (and thus benefit from) the realm of Grace. This passage constitutes both the "next step in our evolution", what "life and evolution now ask of us", and what is essential in order to survive and thrive in the 21st Century!

By so doing, we shall also finally be able to answer the truly fundamental questions of life and of the human condition and it will be at this point that we will, at last, be able to LIVE rather than merely *existing*, to say a big "YES" to Life and live in a conscious rather than unconscious way; namely, to live as adults in a responsible, autonomous, productive, healthy, moral, creative and joyful way! It will also be at this point that we will finally become aware of the fact that, even though life on earth is filled with paradoxes, contradictions, apparent injustices, and appearing as an endless sea of confusion, disorder, trials, tribulations and sufferings, it is truly WORTH LIVING . . . as it constitutes one of the greatest gifts that our Maker gave us!

Chapter VI

QUINTESSENTIAL CHRISTIANITY

The word « quintessence » is fascinating and has a very interesting etymology. It comes from *quinta essentia* which are Latin words meaning the fifth essence or the substance from which the world and man was made. Thus, there is an essence of the physical dimension (Earth), of the emotional dimension (Water), of the mental dimension (Air), and of the spiritual dimension (Fire). Finally comes the "fifth essence" or "quintessence" which is the root, sum, and synthesis of these (Ether). What I mean by the "quintessence of Christianity" is thus what is **truly essential**: its *core, root and substance*. What fundamental role and contribution can that aspect of Christianity make to the new century and millennium we are now entering and why are these truly *since qua non* for our survival and wellbeing in this crucial historical period? These are the fundamental questions I plan to raise, reflect upon, and discuss with you in the present chapter.

First, I want to make a biographical digression and present a very important insight that underlies the present discussion. When I was young I traveled a good deal as my parents took me to different countries and culture. Thus, I was exposed to a multicultural and multiethnic scene at a very difficult time in human history, W.W.II and its aftermath. My first fundamental realization, one that hit me like the proverbial "ton of bricks" was that Life on Earth is an *infinite ocean of pain, suffering and misery!* Everywhere I went, and all the people I met, in one fashion or another and on one level or another, were afflicted by a number of "injustices, personal tragedies, illnesses, persecutions, frustrations, and misery"!

My first reaction to this was "this must really be hell!" What have we done do deserve this and to be born in this infernal world? Thus, the myth of "Paradise Lost" and of "Original Sin" really spoke to me in a very direct and personal, albeit childish way! My second and more pondered reaction was: What are suffering, its nature, roots, dynamics, manifestations and consequences? And my final and most important reaction was: What *can we do about this?* Can we somehow diminish and alleviate this incredible burden of human suffering?

I began my long search and investigation of this truly fundamental question by looking at various social institutions and forms of human knowledge. Specifically, I looked at economics, politics, education, and finally religion, as I mentioned in the first part of this work. Until I came upon the "esoteric" dimension of religion, in general, and of Christianity, in particular, there seemed to be no solution to the universal and age-old problem of human suffering and confusion. Many people and many social institutions purported to deal with them and to offer valid solutions, but none *really worked* and produced truly satisfying results. As I considered the "esoteric" side of religion and the "religion of the Saints and Sages" in particular I did find was I was looking for—the *cognitive perspective* or theoretical framework and the *basic instruments* that were required. But I also found that a great deal of personal work, preparation, and . . . reaching a certain level of consciousness and being were *absolutely essential* for this.

Surely economic well-being, a good political constitution and an honest and competent government, education, science and research *are important* and can contribute a great deal to human wellbeing and evolution, but it cannot contribute what is *truly essential!* "Institutional religion", the outer religion of the people, is also very important and can make valuable contributions but, being inevitably a function of the level of consciousness and being of a person, it cannot touch that which is truly essential. For that you need "quintessential religion", the *Hagia Sophia*, the *Philosophia Perennis*, or the *Wisdom of the Ages* which is only given to the few, the true initiates, Saints, Sages and Prophets of all humanity! What you need is religion being interpreted from the *soul level* and not only from the *personality level!*

Lastly, I am presently convinced (and have been for more than 20 years) that we are living at a very particular, pivotal historical juncture, which we can call the "Apocalypse", "Kali Yuga", the "Great Purification" or the "End of Times". The essence of our historical period is that the very best and the very worst, the greatest dangers and the greatest opportunities, "heaven and hell" as it were, are literally becoming more accessible to ever more people. Its distinguishing feature is the "crisis of adolescence", the passage from "childhood to adulthood", the "High School Graduation" wherein we are forced to raise our level of consciousness, **activate our intuition** and **awaken our spiritual consciousness** . . . as the 21st Century "will either be spiritual or will not be" as André Malraux aptly put it more than 40 years ago!

In essence, practically and specifically, this means that life will become evermore complex, evermore difficult, making greater and greater demands upon each person that could easily lead to more and more *stress* and thus illness, confusion, demoralization, depression, exhaustion, and collapse! If we are to survive and thrive in the 21st Century, we necessarily need to discover, train and be able to utilize our higher faculties, energies and potentialities. The "black box of reason and the senses" which has dominated science and education for the last 300 years at least will simply not be enough! Without genuine intuition and inspiration, without awakening authentic spiritual consciousness, without a conscious and alive connection with something greater than our ego, personality, and the world—without the charisma of the Spirit—we are simply not going to make it! Hence, this question has truly become a question of "life and death" as Life and Evolution are now telling us (in the words of Pitirim Sorokin): *rise to a higher level of consciousness and culture or perish at your own hands!*

And this brings us to *religion* and its two faces, *exoteric* (outer and of the people) and *esoteric* (inner and of the Initiates, Saints, Sages and Prophets) which are unavoidable as we do not all function on the same level of consciousness and being (see the image of the Human Skyscraper and the analogy of the vertical Axis of Consciousness). Tradition itself always recognized and taught that religion has a "letter" which is given and transmitted by the scribes and clergy and a "spirit" which is given and radiated by the Prophets, Saints and Sages (those who function on a higher level of consciousness having reached the threshold of the soul and awakened their spiritual consciousness). Prophets (Saints and Sages) were thus essential in every generation to "vivify the letter by the spirit" and to reinterpret the scriptures and teachings of religion for the level of consciousness, being, and evolution reached by the people and the clergy of a given era.

My central thesis here is quite simple: we have reached the point where tribal religion must now transform itself into a universal religion, where the exoteric and esoteric aspects of religion, the inner and outer aspects, must be recognized and integrated, and where Prophets, Saints and Sages must appear to provide the essential theoretical framework or *perspective* and the practical tools or *instruments* by which we can know, contact, and draw upon the higher energies, laws, and faculties of our being—reconnect with the essence of Reality, both inner and outer—or find *union with God,* as this was known in religion and tradition. It is here that "quintessential Christianity" becomes truly crucial . . . and which has prompted me to write the present chapter.

At a very early age and for the rest of my life, I was introduced to the esoteric aspect of religion in general and of Christianity in particular, due to my own direct personal experiences and the Saints and Sages I met and who provided the perspective and tools, the "keys of reading and interpretation" that I needed. Let me thus state my personal vision, conception, and understanding of Christianity which I found corroborated by the Catholic tradition and expressed in much better words by St. Augustine and the gist of which is the following: *"Christianity is not a new religion; its has always existed and will always exist in that it is the essence of all religions and wisdom traditions expressed in very simple and living words"!*

To be sure Christianity is also a religion, a religion which today has three main branches and a variety of interpretations, implications and applications, but it also contains in its core and essence the *Hagia Sophia*, the *Philosophia Perennis*, the Ageless Wisdom. A simple way of looking at this and explaining this "paradox" is to say that Christianity, like all religions, is a trinity: it implies and has a *body*, a *soul*, and a *spirit*. The "body" is comprised of the New Testament, the Catholic tradition, with its symbols, archetypes, icons, rites and rituals. Its "soul" is the interpretations, implications and applications given to these teachings, symbols, archetypes, icons, rites and rituals. Whereas the "spirit" is the "Life, Power and Wisdom" that can be contacted and received when the body is vivified by its soul which then leads the person to "Live the Life"!

Briefly put, I have come to make the following associations which shed a great deal of light about Christianity and its present threefold manifestation as Eastern Orthodoxy, Roman Catholicism, and Anglo-Saxon Protestantism. Eastern Orthodoxy embodies the "spirit" of the Christian religion, has sought to preserve what the Early Christian and Fathers of the Church, Who were Initiates, have taught, and is most "in line" with what the spiritual tradition has always taught and is linked with John. Roman Catholicism embodies the "soul" of Christianity, its rational and philosophical expression, and is linked with Peter. Protestantism, on the other hand, represents the "body" of Christianity", its most secular, modern and active form, and is linked with Paul. Thus properly understood, they can all complement and complete each other.

The fundamental "sources" for my work and philosophy come from three basic sources that all blend into a forth one: at the spiritual level, the *Spiritual Tradition*, at the religious level, *Eastern Orthodoxy* and the *Catholic Tradition*, and at the psychological level, *Psychosynthesis* which, properly integrated, gave me a background and a way to explain my *own personal experiences*. I owe a great debt of gratitude to many people who have guided me and helped me along the way but in particular to Kyriacos Markides and his two works, *The Mountain of Silence* (Doubleday, 2003) and *Gift of the Desert* (Doubleday, 2005) for his most simple, clear and essential presentation of the essence of the Eastern Orthodox tradition.

My personal involvement with "quintessential Christianity" is a long story which I am not going to recall at this point for lack of time. Suffice it to say that it provided two things for me: first a *theoretical framework* that could explain both my personal, unusual experiences as a child, and what we are presently going through and why we are going through it; second, *practical instruments* to help me to recover my health, which was essential for me to accomplish my work and destiny when the best medical authorities told me that this was not possible.

While the cognitive, philosophical aspect was important and interesting, it was the second aspect, the practical healing, that was truly *essential and life-determining* for me. In a nutshell, I desperately needed help without which a "meaningful life" would be over for me. I also realized and lived, in my own being and life, the famous saying of Angelus Silesius that contains the substance of the esoteric aspect of religion: "Should Christ be born a thousand times in Bethlehem but not in my own soul, I would still be lost!" Thus, I believe that the model that I experienced and lived has a larger use and importance for all of us who are alive in the 21st Century and who are also confronted with very difficult challenges! So what is "quintessential Christianity" what is its role at our present time and what can it do for us at a very simple and practical level?

Quintessential Christianity is not "another religion" rather it is the *substance and essence*, the very heart and core, of all *authentic religions*. It has always existed and will always exist as long as there are evolving human beings on this earth. It is what I like to call the "Spiritual Tradition", the *Hagia Sophia*, and *Philosophia Perennis* or Ageless Wisdom. As such, it can provide us with a blue print or cognitive perspective that can show us:

- Who and what we are, our true identity.
- Where we come from, our origins.
- Where we are going, our destiny.
- Why we were born in this world, our vocation.
- Where we are at the present time and what we are called to do, our evolutionary duty.
- Hence, it can help us answer the "Riddle of the Sphinx", the next great step and challenge in our becoming and evolution.
- Then, it can also show us Who and what are God, Life, the Universe, good and evil, the *condition humaine*.

But it is also more than the above, a compendium of essential human knowledge and understanding that helps us to *reconcile opposites* and explain the paradoxes and contradictions that characterize the human condition. It is also a set of practical means by which we can consciously participate in perfecting ourselves and accomplishing our true destiny by establishing the right relationship with ourselves (the microcosm) and with God (the macrocosm). Finally and most important, it is also a *living source of Love* which gives us the motivation and desire to live and realize the foregoing. It is what can lead us, by degree to the inexhaustible and living Source of Life, Love, and Wisdom that exists both within ourselves and in the universe and which tradition called "God".

What was the truly fundamental or "essential task" of Jesus Christ? It was to talk about, bring, and life three fundamental things:

- *"The Kingdom of God"*, which is what I would call *spiritual consciousness* that we must now achieve if we are to survive and thrive in the 21st Century. Jesus rightfully said, "Seek ye first the Kingdom of God and its righteousness, and all these things shall be added unto you". But it is perhaps only **now** that we can truly understand what that means and appreciate its role and importance.
- *"The Gifts of the Holy Spirit"*, the various charismas that we all have potentially and now must develop and be able to access. These involve all the parapsychological and psychic powers we have discovered and some that we have not yet discovered but which involve higher laws, principles and energies than those that our science is aware of and which we already have, but at a *potential* and not yet at an *actual* level! Moreover, it implies using them to do *God's Will* and not the *will of our own ego*, which is a most important distinction!
- An *Archetype* and *Prototype* of what we can and will become when we fulfill our destiny and have actualized all of our faculties and potentialities and realized our spiritual Self. As we have reached the point where our evolution becomes conscious, we must *consciously* perfect and complete our being and this requires an "ideal model" to work towards . . .

The core axiom of the Eastern Orthodox Church is that "God became Man so that Man can become God" which was first enunciated by St. Athanasios and which beautifully epitomized both the role and goal of Christianity and that of human beings. Thus, the Orthodox Tradition presented and emphasized the following core concepts and insights as carried forward by the Monks of Mount Athos, the *Gerontikon* or Elders, and the Saints and Sages:

1. The central axis of the authentic spiritual life is defined by two core concepts, *askesis* and *ecclesia*, or spiritual exercises and an intentional group or "spiritual family" (which is the Christian equivalent of the Buddhist *Upaya* and *Santsang*); followed by the *love of God* or **prayer** (on the vertical axis) and the *love of our fellows humans* or **service** (on the horizontal axis).
2. Where we are coming from and where we are going, together with where we now are and what constitutes our present crucial evolutionary task, is beautifully described by the parable of the *Prodigal Son*. We are all the "Solar Hero" or the "Prodigal Son". We came from the spiritual worlds to the physical one to eventually return to the spiritual worlds and our Source and Essence. Now we have reached the crucial "crossroads" where involution (the descent of spirit into matter) has to turn into evolution (the ascent back of matter into spirit). Hence, the "crisis of adolescence" or the Apocalypse!

3. Because of the Fall we now live in a state of *amartia* (which is the Greek work for "sin" but which has very different connotations and denotations). It means, essentially, to have forgotten our purpose, having "missed our target" and *derailed ourselves* by cutting ourselves off from God and His Love. Thus the essential illness of our times is the *illness of the heart*, of love, and of the love of God in particular.

4. The Ecclesia is a "clinic" with trained physicians and therapists which can help us "open our hearts", remove its pathologies, and reconnect us with God and His Love. The pathologies of the heart, according to this tradition, are: *ignorance* of God, *forgetfulness* of God and ourselves, hardening of the heart or *hardness* (lack of feeling and compassion), *blindness* (losing sight and sensibility to the Uncreated Light) and *contamination* (seeking the glamour and pleasures of the world). The essential remedy to "open the human heart to the Uncreated Light" is to *crush the heart,* as the Elders and the Saints teach that "God will never spurn a broken heart". This is why they ask God to "begin breaking the granite, to crush their heart!" This is also the reason why suffering, perceived and experienced in the proper way, can be very positive and redeeming because it is what breaks the heart . . . achieving the same thing but in an opposite way as true love.

5. To return to God (both within and without our selves) we need to *repent,* change our ways, which we call *conversion* or in Greek *metanoia* (which again, has different connotations and denotations). Metanoia then opens the way to *Catharsis, Fotisis,* and *Theosis* which is the essential "threefold way" back to God.

6. Catharsis implies *purification* of the heart and *consecration* of the will. This in time will lead to Fotisis.

7. Fotisis is *illumination,* the descent of the Light into the heart of man (into his "energy-bodies, his Tree of Life and its psychospiritual centers). This is the response of grace to the human efforts directed to God to complete the Great Work of human regeneration.

8. Theosis implies *deification,* union with God, becoming one with God, hence becoming a "Christed human being" which is our final destination. This occurs when we have created a "temple" or "church" for Christ in our souls and hearts so that He can be born, grow, operate and become resurrected **in us** (in our energy—bodies, our Tree of Life and its psychospiritual centers). This is our fabulous destiny and what we have come to achieve in this world and which was made possible by the Incarnation of Christ in our world!

In simple, practical and concrete words, what does all of this mean and how can we profit from it? First, and this is most important as we are living in a relative world, we should be careful and choose accurately our basic "yardstick-model" or "frame of reference": we should study *Saints, Sages, and spiritually awakened* persons rather than *normal or sick persons* if we want to understand human nature, our origins and destiny, and what we have come to do in this world; then, we should study *health and life* rather than *pathology* and *dead-matter* when it comes to health-care and medicine. We should study the early Christian Communities and the monks of Mount Athos who took Jesus Christ, the God-Man and fully actualized Person as their essential "Model" and who demonstrated that *"peace profound"* that passeth human understanding" and which is the seal of attainment and authenticity for all religions.

More than various gifts and charismas (such as clairvoyance, prophecy, being able to read through the human soul, precognition, retro-cognition, levitation, out-of-the-body experiences, and the gift of healing, spiritual, psychological and physical, etc.), it was the *love they had for God and for one another*, the ability to remain joyful, serene and non-violent in the most difficult and painful situations that characterized them and which can serve a splendid ideal and model for us today. It was their recognition that Light and Good are greater than Darkness and Evil, that there is no human experience from which we cannot learn something and benefit from . . . provided the Light of God is with us! It was their ability to keep hope in adversity and to transform adversity in opportunity.

So, we should live today in an *impeccable way*, dedicating all that we do to God, the Uncreated Light and the inexhaustible and living Source of Life, Love, and Wisdom, always doing our best, not less but not more either! We should seek to unite our *human efforts* with *grace*, the male and female polarities, spirit and matter, the inner and the outer. We should remember that it is **love**, not knowledge and power (important as these are) that is most important thus expressing love in all our relationships and realizing that "what we do unto others, ultimately we do unto ourselves". We should learn to **accept** whatever Life (and our destiny) brings to us and transform it into a *spiritual exercise* for our own growth and self-actualization. And this will enable us to exorcize and banish the most real and dangerous of "devils": fear, anxiety, resentment, jealousy, envy, and greed enabling us to face and cope with whatever we shall be confronted with and whatever challenge will come our way. For then we shall have substituted "essential wealth" ("spiritual "gold") for "secondary wealth" (money and physical gold)!

As I already mentioned before, the religion of the future, of the 21st Century in particular will have to be a *universal religion* with a sound *metaphysical foundation* and with *practical instruments* whereby we can understand Who we really are, what we have come to do in this world, where we now stand in our evolution, what is our next crucial step in becoming and how we can achieve our glorious destiny! Hence, it will have to reconcile and blend the "letter" with the "spirit", its exoteric with its esoteric aspect and the religion of the people with that of the Saints and Sages! To achieve this, we need to reach our "spiritual puberty" where we substitute God to the world, spiritual to worldly aspirations and where we move from the personality to the soul level!

This has always been done by some. Several persons are now working towards this and eventually we will all have to do in that this is what constitutes God's Plan for us, for His Children! This is also what the true *spiritual adventure*, the greatest and most important adventure of them all is all about and **now** is the time to live it! Since the essential problem of the human condition is the **problem of love**, we now need to accomplish three basic transformations or *metanoia*: *learn how to transform an enemy into a friend, a parasite into a saprophyte, and a demon into an angel*—learn, in other words, how to **truly love** for this is what will redeem both ourselves and the world with the united human and divine forces!

Chapter VII

THE NEW ENCYCLOPEDIA, A COMPENDIUM OF HUMAN KNOWLEDGE FOR THE 21ST CENTURY

As we are entering the new Millennium and beginning the 21st century there is a very urgent need for something quite old and important: reconcile *analysis* (which seeks to break things down into smaller and smaller parts and to penetrate ever deeper into the microcosm) and *synthesis* (which seeks to relate things into larger and larger whole and to penetrate ever further into the macrocosm); that is to relate and coordinate human knowledge into a rational and intelligible whole where all the parts are linked and interacting with each other in a *meaningful* fashion. In other words, this means to relate religion, science and philosophy into a larger more integral and holistic whole which recognizes and integrates the *spiritual dimension* . . . which may well be the "missing" cornerstone and capstone of this masterful endeavor!

Three questions immediately come to mind: Is this possible and feasible? And, if so, how and has it ever been attempted before? How can we put together, connect and interrelate all of the incredibly complex, multidimensional, and contradictory elements of the world and fragments of our own being and consciousness? Human communication, after the "Tower of Babel" (a fascinating symbol and archetype with several levels of interpretations and different meanings), is certainly not an easy process. Most people do not communicate or communicate only in fragmentary, dissociated, and contradictory ways. They do not agree and can perceive, define, and react to the *same thing* in very different ways. Paradoxes, contradictions, and opposites abound in our world and all human and academic disciplines are filled with different and even opposed theories and explanations which are constantly being "redefined", "refined" and "amplified".

Historically speaking, however, we can find two very interesting insights: First, this is not a new or untried endeavor, it has, in fact, been attempted and proposed all along our known human history with varying results and success. Second, it was said, already more than 2,000 years ago, and repeated along the way, by the most evolved and brightest persons, to: "seek ye first the "Kingdom of God" (i.e. spiritual consciousness) and all of these things shall be added unto you" (that is, what is important for you). Now, in our fragmented, alienated, polluted, and violent world where millions kill each other, die of starvation, live lives of "quiet desperation", or are tortured by various physical and psychological diseases which keep mutating and multiplying each other, and where *depression* and *alienation* may well be one of the most important explanatory factors, this "compendium of human knowledge" is *very important*, particularly at this *historical juncture!*

Deeply imbedded in human nature and in the depths of our human consciousness, lies a truly perennial and universal need and aspiration: that of being able to understand and find meaning and significance in what we are and what we live, or for authentic *knowledge!* Equally important, universal and perennial, are also the need for *love* and for *life*, for feeling, desiring and appreciating, for motivation, and for vital and creative energies, for power, but these will be discussed and analyzed at another time and in another context. It has been rightfully said that "if man can understand and find meaning, significance and value in what he is living through, he can go through anything without cracking up!" Thus, a school of psychotherapy has emerged, *logotherapy*, which seeks to heal various pathologies by seeking for *personal meaning . . .* and whose motto is "so long as man has a *why*, he can bear any *how*".

Given our historical juncture, the level of human consciousness, being and evolution we have reached and the present transformational crisis we are faced with, (our "crisis of adolescence" and the "High School graduation exam" that is before us), we need a "hermeneutic key", a "software program", to understand and make sense of ourselves and of the world in which we live. We need to be able to understand who we are, why we came into this world, what we can and what we cannot do, and what is the goal or purpose of the human adventure and condition; we also need to be able to understand the sociocultural world in which we live, its distinctive characteristics and present trends. I am convinced that the *spiritual tradition* and the emerging *spiritual science* can provide us with precisely that "key and program" and the presently "missing link"!

Without them, life could become quite demoralizing, bleak and meaningless; we could very easily reach the point where we would no longer want or be able to cope with the rising challenges of our times and give up on life. We could become quite depressed and seek a number of addictions to escape a "reality" that appears more and more paradoxical, unjust, and worthless. We could easily come to the conscious or unconscious conclusion that evil is greater than good, that we are hopelessly alienated and helpless to change our situation, that we are alone in the world and left to our own devices which have bread the cancer-man rather than the God-Man, and thus seek to destroy ourselves, or the world, in a direct or indirect way.

With them, we could come to the opposite conclusion while not denying any of the negative aspects that are present, but reframing them in a larger and more positive framework. We could understand how we got to where we are today, what is the true nature of our present situation and what we can realistically do about it. We could get the perspective and the instruments to allow us to cope with the present and coming challenges and especially to *want to do this* and to really *give the very best we have to this endeavor* by understanding its deeper meaning and significance and by becoming aware that it is definitely and unquestionably WORTH IT, even under the most difficult and painful circumstances!

Looking now at the unfoldment of human history and of the biography of ideas we find some very interesting and revealing facts. All primitive and traditional societies and cultures had a theoretical and practical *synthesis of knowledge* woven around religion and the sacred. Briefly put, their form of government was essentially a *theocracy* where the ruling elite were Sages or counseled by Sages. Priests and Kings were Sages or counseled by Sages, and thus a *practical wisdom* existed and ensured the survival of the individual and of the group. This corresponded to the "infancy" of humanity where most people were "babies" or "children" who needed parents, elders, and sages to take care of them, protect them and tell them what do. During that phase *instinct* and then *tradition* was king! People did not think too much, they had to survive and go on and for that *obedience* and *compliance* with the values and norms set by the ruling elite were essential.

This state of affairs prevailed roughly until the end of the Middle Ages and up to the Renaissance. In the West, religion provided the unifying cement for theology, anthropology, and cosmology, and their interrelations. Philosophy provided the glue that brought together what we knew about God, Man, and the Universe, but philosophy was dominated by religion which imposed its own basic world-view, dogmas, and priorities. Then, the unthinkable occurred: the dominance and hold of religion was broken (essentially because of the corruption of its elite who were sinking deeper and deeper into egoism, despotism, and hedonism and because of the rising consciousness of people who wanted and demanded more) and was replaced by *science* which was made possible by the discovery and adoption of the *scientific method*.

The scientific method, in essence, substituted *tradition and authority* by direct *personal observation and experience*. This means essentially that instead of citing a tradition or quoting an expert, now one had to reach one's own personal observations and experiences which would become possible when one followed the same set of rules and procedures. Now if one had to be able to see or experience something, measure it and quantify it, and make it repeatable for others who were trained in the same fashion and who played by the same rules, this had a profound impact on what we called "reality" and "truth". And this impact was double: it greatly restricted "reality" and "truth", bringing them down to their lowest common denominator . . . or almost, but it also made that "reality" and "truth" far more "alive" and "meaningful" as it became a "personal and lived thing"!

Thus about four-five centuries ago the existing "compendium of human knowledge", with its concomitant "consensus", began to break down. Science replaced religion, cosmology became the natural sciences which splintered and multiplied; anthropology became the human or natural sciences which also splintered and multiplied; and finally theology became more and more anemic, losing its former prestige and power, and was relegated to religion and its various expressions and denominations. Analysis prevailed over synthesis and "having" over "being", scientific knowledge replaced wisdom with the final objective of giving us *power*, power over nature and over others! We literally "conquered the physical world" but "lost our own soul" in the process. Alienation, fragmentation, confusion, conflict, demoralization and depression set in which led to a truly suicidal course of action insofar as both the *world* (the environment) and *ourselves* (our health and well being) were concerned.

To continue the image and analogy I had used earlier, this phase of human evolution truly corresponds to the period of "adolescence". While babies and children need parents, someone to protect them, keep them alive, guide them and tell them what to do, adolescents rebel against all of this and want *independence*; they want to discover who they are and what are their limits, and thus they reject tradition, their parents, former authorities, and want to *experiment with everything* . . . to have their own personal experiences and reach their conclusions. In the process, however, as the world and human nature are extremely complex and multidimensional, they may intervene and do things which have great *unknowns* and *imponderables* and which consequences they cannot anticipate, but that they will have to assume and to live with! And, to my mind, this is what best describes our present historical period!

Our present historical period (specifically from the end of World War II to the end of the first half of the 21st century or from 1950 to 2050) is characterized by a tremendous transformation and transition, a true *metanoia* of our level of consciousness, values, and priorities. It is the period in which the greatest dangers but also the greatest opportunities, the very best and the very worst, "heaven and hell", as it were, become accessible to an ever-growing number of persons. It is also the period where *choice* becomes more and more important in that if we choose and take the *ascending spiral* our lives can improve dramatically; but, were we to choose and take the *descending spiral* we could easily destroy ourselves, our environment and others.

This is why this period has been called the Apocalypse, the Kali Yuga, the time of the Great Purification and other such names. I choose to view it as our "adolescence" characterized by our "High School Graduation" or "Maturity Exam". The essential trait of this period is very simple: we need to raise our level of consciousness and being and to access higher energies, laws, and principles . . . or we will not make it into the 21st Century! Put another way, "the 21st Century will either *be spiritual* . . . or will *not be*!" as it is "spiritual consciousness" (which used to be called the "Kingdom of God") that we need to develop and utilize to meet the growing challenges now thrown by Life and Evolution to the human spirit.

Thus, if we succeed in *activating our intuition* and *awakening our spiritual consciousness*, not only we will "make it" but we will enter a far better and more meaningful period that we have ever had! And it will be our intuition and spiritual consciousness that will lead us to bring about that new "encyclopedia", or compendium of human knowledge, that will give meaning, purpose and value to the manifold and growing areas of human experience and knowledge. To do this I believe that we need a *spiritual science*, just like we developed a natural and social science, and it is this "spiritual science" which I see as now emerging and providing the solution to the fundamental human problems.

To look at it from a different angle, Joachim da Flores, a brilliant Italian thinker, philosopher and mystic (like Dante Alighieri or Giordano Bruno) said a long time something that is very interesting and which could explain many things. He said that religion essentially went through three basic phases: the *religion of the Father*, focused on *knowledge*, the *religion of the Son*, focused on *love*, and the *religion of the Holy Spirit* focused on a *full realization and integration* of the former. In a sense, we could say that the "religion of the Father" was that given to "babies and children"; the religion of the Son was that given to "children, adolescents and young adults" and the religion of the Holy Spirit that which will be given to "young and mature adults". And this for a very good reason!

The religion of the Holy Spirit is that of the full realization and integration of the promises made by the former stages, hence it gives real and incredible powers. But these powers must be used with *wisdom* and *maturity*, and with *love*, lest they create real catastrophes for all involved. Since we have reached our "adolescent stage" and began to systematically develop scientific knowledge and create more sophisticated "toys" and powers, we have gotten a great deal more *power* than we ever had before. And we are still developing and increasing that power by learning how to harness the latent powers of the mind and will. With this power we have created evermore sophisticated and powerful weapons, machines, and drugs which threaten to destroy the equilibrium of the world, the homeostasis of our bodies and psyches, and thus destroy not only our "enemies" but also ourselves and the very world in which we live!

Looked at from yet another angle, we can find in our universal symbolism, myths and fairy tales a fundamental point that leads us to the same conclusion. A young *prince*, the son of a king and queen, will someday awaken a *princess*, the child of a king and queen, who had fallen asleep *with a kiss*! In universal symbolism, the "king" always represented spirit, the "queen" nature or matter, the prince extraverted consciousness or *science* and the princess introverted consciousness or our *soul*! So what does this universal myth tell us? It tells us that when science will have reached a certain stage and level and when it will rediscover and integrate **love**, it will help us rediscover our soul and make it come alive . . . And, obviously, I believe that this time is our present historical period!

One thing, however, is very clear and definite: if we want to continue to live and evolve, if we want to find truly satisfying answers to the fundamental problems, needs and aspirations, of our times, we have to **raise our level of consciousness and being**—we have to *activate our intuition* and *awaken our spiritual consciousness*. Now this transformation and expansion of human consciousness cannot occur by more study, research and the further development of our minds just as it cannot be brought about by our human efforts alone! It can only occur when we link the mind with the heart, when logos and eros, knowledge and love, are fused so that we can give birth to *wisdom*; when the male principle has recognized and integrated the female principle and when human effort is completed by divine grace.

We could continue our academic and scientific studies utilizing only our senses, reason, and imagination for centuries, millennia, and even millions of years but our human efforts alone would never lead us and enable us to activate our spiritual consciousness! Just like the mind and the heart must be brought together by the will at the human and personality level, so human effort and divine grace must also be brought together at the soul level so as to reawaken our souls and activate both our intuition and our spiritual consciousness. This clearly involves a major *metanoia* or inversion, and a great deal of personal work, humility, and receptivity. What it involves, essentially, is the fusion of "form" and "force", of the "temple" with its Tenant, of Man with God.

If we look at knowledge in a broader sense, we can see that it is the product of two great and opposed forces: those that come from *ourselves*, from our human nature, and those that come from *something Else* that is greater than ourselves, from the "creature' and from the "Creator". Knowledge, therefore, has always been "natural" and "revealed"; *natural knowledge* being gathered through our efforts and the use of our human faculties and *revealed knowledge* coming down the planes and interdimensionally from a greater Source than our own. Until now these two forms of knowledge have been at odds with each other and even opposed each other . . . which is the reason why it is said in the Holy Scriptures that "the wisdom of God is foolishness in the eyes of men and the wisdom of men is foolishness in the eyes of God".

In essence, the "wisdom of God", revealed knowledge, is that which integrates and seeks the *good of the whole* which, for human beings, means that which brings *peace* and preserves *harmony*; whereas the "wisdom of men", natural knowledge, is that which focuses upon and seeks the *good of the part* which, for human beings, means that which brings *conflict* and creates *disharmonies*. Moreover, the "wisdom of men" is well described by Freud's reality principle which states that "men seek pleasure and try to avoid pain" which means, in simple words, that they will strive to make their lives ever more predictable, comfortable and filled with pleasures! The "wisdom of God", on the other hand, implies essentially to grow, to evolve, to actualize our potentialities and realize our Self—to become more than what we are! Unfortunately, we cannot achieve this goal in this world without efforts, sacrifices, taking risks and suffering.

To move on to this new level of consciousness and being, to awaken our spiritual consciousness, several things are required. First, there are certain basic assumptions that must be made, developed, and integrated. Second, we must also live a certain type of life where everything becomes important as everything is related to everything else. Hence, a major "transformation" and "turning around" or *metanoia*, conversion, is required. We shall now briefly look at these two respectively:

Core assumptions and presuppositions, ideas and insights

To bring about this major transformation and new encyclopedia that corresponds to the "adult" period of our evolution there are certain points: presuppositions, intuitions, and core ideas that are truly fundamental and that are worth discussing clearly and stating explicitly. These are:

1. *A theory of human nature*: basic assumptions about the anatomy and physiology of our being. What are we, what are we made of, where do we come from, where are we going, and what are we meant to accomplish in this world both at the essential, overall level, and at the specific present moment and cycle?
2. *A model of the psyche*: basic assumptions about the nature, structure, functions, dynamics, and contributions of our human consciousness. What can human consciousness do and what can it not do for us?
3. *An epistemology*: what constitutes true and valid knowledge? How do we get it and verify it? Can we change and expand it not only quantitatively but also qualitatively?
4. *As we live in the world of duality and relativity, what is our basic "reference point"?* Is it the earth, our solar system, our galaxy? Is it a static or a dynamic system in motion? Is it single parts or parts in interaction with other parts in various "systems"? And when it comes to

human beings, is it "normal persons", "sick persons", or Saints, Sages, and spiritually awakened persons who have realized higher states of consciousness, faculties, and energies? Is it Life and alive systems or is it dead parts and systems?

The above constitute truly essential questions that we must all raise. Depending on we answer them, we will reach very different conclusions, values and priorities. And, depending on our level of consciousness and being, there are very different ways of answering them as "reality" and "truth" are truly functions of our level of consciousness and being. Then, come the truly core insights and mother-ideas of the spiritual tradition and perspective which are:

- *The human sky-scraper and "vertical axis of consciousness*: While we all live in the same biophysical and sociocultural world, we do not all function on the same level of consciousness and being and thus we will perceive define and react to the same thing in very different ways. While there are 7 possible levels of consciousness (and thus types of person), 4 are the ones that are truly practical and "operational" as the other 3 are still very rare.
- *The microcosm-macrocosm analogy*: A human being is truly the synthesis of all there is and thus contains a part of nature (the physical body), a part of humanity (the psyche) and a part of God (the Pneuma, spirit, or divine spark). Thus, there is nothing outside of us which is not also inside of us and vice versa.
- *"Only like can know like"*: This is an old hermetic and alchemical axiom but which is very true and important. It essentially claims that one can only recognize and interact with something which he already has *within his own being*. Thus to know God you need to activate the part of God you have within your own nature; for, according to the principle of resonance and consonance, we could never perceive or make exchanges with something that was truly alien to our being and which lacked a corresponding part in it.
- *The nature, functions, and dynamics of symbolic and analytical language* which is quite different and in some ways opposed to descriptive and analytical language which we use in everyday speech and in science. The first is dynamic and ever-unfolding, being related to our level of consciousness and being and to our personal experiences and values, while the latter is static and set once and for all.
- *The parable of the Prodigal Son*: which tells us who we are, where we are coming from, where we are going, and what point we have reached in our long pilgrimage through the world of matter. It describes, analogically and in symbols, the process of *involution* (the descent

of spirit into matter) and of *evolution* (the ascent of matter back into spirit) and of the crucial "turning point" where involution has to turn into evolution . . . which is *now*, our present historical period!

- *The essential role and nature of love and of relationships.* This in all areas of human endeavor including the process of *knowing itself.* The essential process by which we grow and evolve, by which we actualize our faculties and potentialities, and by which we become more than what we are, is *interaction*, the law of exchange or give and take.

- *The process by which we can transform and raise our level of consciousness and being.* This is done by learning how to open ourselves and by learning how to *love*, giving and receiving, both on the vertical and on the horizontal level. It involves the love of God (prayer) and the love of our fellow humans (service) which then brings about the love of ourselves, of nature, and of Life!

- *The law of reincarnation or rebirth.* It is literally impossible for a human being to fulfill his destiny and to achieve his perfection in one life time, even if it lasted 120 years which is our biological limit and which few can reach. A much longer period of time is necessary for us to go through all the experiences we need to actualize all of our faculties and potentialities and to learn all the lessons of the physical plane. Were we to have only one shot on earth, which would decide our existence in eternity, this would make a mockery of *divine justice* and an incredible *waste of potentialities* which would be absurd! Thus we have multiple lives on earth which are as many as is necessary for us to learn all our earthly lessons and to fulfill the purpose for which we were created.

- *Its corollary principle of karma, of action and reaction.* This simply means that we shall, indeed, "reap what we sawed", that what we do unto others we do unto ourselves; that the incredible diversity and apparent "injustices" that are quite obvious in human experience is not a "punishment" or the work of "random chance", luck or misfortune, but another "learning opportunity" to discover what we like and want or not and the consequences of what we are choosing and doing! All religions, especially in their mystical expression, and all spiritual traditions recognized and taught the principle of reincarnation and of karma, in one fashion or another in a more or less explicit fashion. In the Western traditions, these two principles have always been part of the Mysteries that were not given to all but only to those in the "Upper Chamber", to the initiates who had been properly trained and who were mature enough to receive them and use them wisely.

- *The fact that the mortal may attain to the knowledge of the spiritual while yet incarnate!* Interestingly enough, we do not have to "die" in order to access to the spiritual world and to the higher levels of consciousness and being. We can and must achieve this while "in the body", or return here until we have achieved it! So it is here, on this plane of being, that we have to find and realize the Great Pearl, the Kingdom of Heaven or spiritual consciousness!

- *The fact that Life is without beginning and without ending in an evolutionary scale of progression.* From this viewpoint, everything that exists is "alive" and "intelligent" or conscious but in very different quantities and qualities. Thus Life can never be destroyed, it can only be changed and transformed.

- Finally that what we call *"Reality"*, both external and internal, in the microcosm (man) or the macrocosm (the universe), *is made up of energies and vibrations that manifest through specific frequencies* that have a practically infinite range of expressions. Thus, it is the principle of "consonance and resonance" or of "only like can know like" that can bring us in touch with specific frequencies that translate as specific states of consciousness and energies. Our true "free will" is thus our ability to "shift frequencies" and, therefore, *levels of consciousness* which make available to us a wide range of "programs" or "possibilities" both on the positive and on the negative end.

The great transition and transformation we are now all living through, as both spectators and actors, and which our soul chose before it incarnate on earth (our "crisis of adolescence" and "maturity exam") demand many basic qualitative changes which few can yet see or understand. When it comes to the process of acquiring knowledge, especially higher knowledge, and to the process of human and spiritual growth, there are certain very basic points and insights that must be understood and lived if we genuinely want to raise our level of consciousness and being and enter into the higher floors of the "human sky-scraper". Briefly put, these are the following:

First, we need to realize that in order to have access to higher states of consciousness and being, hence, to access a more global and profound knowledge (which is not mental or cerebral in nature) we need to **live in a certain way**. Unlike academic, scientific and mental knowledge which can be acquired by certain mental efforts and disciplines (schools, laboratories, and intellectual training) but which leave us free to live our personal lives as we wish; the higher and more integral form of knowledge, which is a blend of natural and revealed knowledge, and which includes the activation of our intuition and the awakening of our spiritual consciousness, demands that we live in a *conscious way*! Namely, that we live in a responsible, autonomous, productive, healthy, moral, creative and joyful way where *absolutely everything* that we think, feel, wish, say and do is *important* . . . as it has an impact on everything else!

In the past and until quite recently, this meant that we had to leave the world and seek the seclusion and protection of a monastery and convent . . . and even then most who sought that kind of life did not achieve that higher knowledge as they may not have been "ready" for it! Today, however, we do not have to leave the world and retire to a secluded and protected environment; we need *to live in the world but not for the world* as it was stated, many times and in many ways, by the spiritual tradition. This in turn means many things, the most important of which are:

1. To live a balanced and harmonious life with the "right measure, the right proportion, the right timing and the right distance", what used to be called and rightly so, the *golden mean*!

2. To cultivate the *cardinal virtues* (hope, faith, charity, patience, perseverance, humility, sobriety) thus diminishing the fundamental vices (fear, guilt, anger, gluttony, despair, cowardness, pride) so as to "make them flesh" and live by them.

3. To develop and integrate the ontological attributes of both God and Man, *knowledge*, *love* and *power* but where the accent is put on **love** which remains primary.

4. To focus upon and privilege what is *eternal* over what is *temporal* (one of the great antidotes for stress, conflict and depression) and thus to "rediscover" and privilege the *vertical dimension* . . . which we have neglected if not abandoned for the horizontal one during the last 500 years at least.

5. To realize that so long as one can *learn* something, *love* someone or something, and *make a difference* (in one's life and that of others), our lives will have meaning, purpose, and value as they will enable us to grow and become more than what we are!

6. To decide and learn how to live in an *impeccable way* so as to develop *character* and *integrity* (which can always be done in all human circumstances and conditions as it is an "inner" and not an "outer" quality) rather than seeking what is expedient or "less painful".

7. To learn how to *forgive*, both ourselves and others, as we are not yet perfect beings but imperfect beings undergoing an evolution, and thus are bound to make mistakes. What Heaven and our higher Self asks of us is not that we be *perfect*, just that we do *the best we can* with what we have, not less but not more either!

8. To understand the proper relationship between *human effort*, what we can and should do, and *divine grace*, what we need to ask for as it does not depend on us, or the marriage of the male and female principles.

9. To learn how to love God through conscious and effective *prayer* and to love our fellow humans through practical and effective *service* and

affection. The strange point here is that the best way to obtain something, on a lasting and meaningful basis, is to make it available to others. To learn that we are all ONE on the higher planes and thus that what one does to others one does to oneself . . . and vice versa!

10. To (slowly and progressively) get to the point where one can truly say (and mean it in one's heart!): "*nihil humanum alienum a me puto*", nothing that is human will be alien or foreign to me; in other words, whatever happened to any human being, for good or for evil, can happen to me, but I will make the effort to learn to live without fear and guilt so that I can truly appreciate and be grateful for all that happens to me.

11. To realize that we all have a *destiny* in this world, something which we came here to do and which our soul "picked" (with the help of higher Beings before we incarnated on earth). Thus that the true secret of happiness and peace is no more and no less than *fulfilling that destiny*, to be true to ourselves and cultivate real integrity, rather than all the things the world tries to make us believe will bring that happiness.

12. Last but not least, to develop the intuitive discernment and judgment to understand that the world is full of *glamour* and *temptations* which it will seek to throw upon us. That Evil, the devil and demons do exist, but that they have a function in creation and that ultimately they also work for the realization of God's ultimate Plan. Hence, that we should *resist them* but not *fear or hate them*! Good exists so that we can say "yes" to it, and evil exits so that we can say "no" to it, as Roberto Assagioli liked to repeat!

At the present time, given our level of consciousness and the point we have reached in our evolution, we have come to a "crossroads" where we are faced with a very major challenge: to become adults and assume both our responsibilities and our privileges. The *rite de passage* between "childhood" and "adulthood" and fraught with dangers and opportunities . . . which can create a great deal of confusion and suffering. But, we have no choice as *grow and evolve* we must and so we have to face our "Apocalypse, "Armageddon", and "maturity exam". One of the basic implications of this is that we must now go through a very important "turn around" or metanoia: *involution* must turn to *evolution*, from focusing on the world and descending further into matter, we must now focus on the spirit by turning inwards and upwards; and our "center of gravity" (basic point of reference and authority) must now turn from the world to our own soul!

This means that our basic values, priorities, and "measuring-rod" must change. One very simple but essential way of looking at this, from a symbolic and archetypal point of view, is to meditate on the famous declaration of Angelus Silesius: "Though Christ a thousand times is born in Bethlehem and not in my own soul, I would still be lost"! In simpler but truly essential terms this means that *I must now live and experience*, within my own being, consciousness and life, all the essential things that happened in the world and in history (which is the true meaning of the microcosm/macrocosm analogy). And as the "old" has not yet died and let go completely and as the "new" is not yet fully born and in control, we are *torn between the two* (between the personality and the soul, the ego and the Self, the outer and the inner) and this is neither pleasant nor easy, but it is necessary!

At the personal level, it creates a great deal of confusion, cynicism, tension and depression while at the social level it creates corruption, demoralization, and the turning of the means into the end and of the part into the whole. Thus, at the micro level, we see and experience a great deal of physical and psychological pathology whereas at the macro level we see all social institutions which are literally "crumbling". People no longer really believe, trust, or respect them. They see them as being a "leviathan" which has grown out of control and which seeks to further its own self-interests by doing the minimum amount of work to fulfill their original mission. Hence, many people do not want to give much to them while they seek to derive as many benefits from them as they can! And this unfortunately, is true of all social institutions: religion, government, health-care, education, the family, etc.

Fortunately, however, there are still many people who have character and integrity and who still hold unto the old values and priorities or the new, emerging ones and who give a great deal of themselves: work, care, and dedication for, without these "just people", society would truly break apart and we would experience the "war of all against all" and live the old Roman adage, "homo homini lupus"! At the individual level we would also crumble "rusting away" with illnesses, depression, egoism, materialism, and nihilism. According to the spiritual tradition, "whenever the darkness is greatest, the light is nearest" for it is in times of *great need* that *great help* comes. At a more concrete level, this means that it is at a time like ours that Great Souls are born into the world to help humankind in its evolution and that God and grace are nearest!

Thus, from the foregoing, we can deduce that religion, science, government, the economy, education, health-care, the family, etc. will have to go through a major redefinition and reorganization. They are all very important to both the individual and to society and are deeply interrelated with each other, but we have to "begin somewhere" and that "somewhere" for me is the institution (s) that touch our ontological qualities which are *knowledge, love,* and *will* (vital and creative energies). In the past, that was *religion* and today it is *science*. Today, I believe that these two can come together, complement each other, and go further than any one could go alone. Moreover, I firmly believe that the time has really for us to achieve this union or synthesis . . . which could well be the "religion of the Holy Spirit" foreseen by Joachim da Flores! Let's now take a closer look.

Religion "comes down from above", it works with *grace*, higher energies and states of consciousness, and utilizes *intuition* and *revelation*. The founders and core "models" of religion are Saints, Sages, Prophets, and spiritually enlightened persons who utilize the right brain hemisphere and the female polarity; of necessity they speak in symbols, archetypes, parables, allegories and myths which are dynamic and unfolding with many different meanings, implications and applications, depending on the level of consciousness and evolution of the persons who are their recipient.

Thus, religion offers not a clear, ready-made, and fixed truth but rather a *mine* and a *treasure* that must be *used* and *lived*. As a result, there are really 4 basic levels of interpretation, implication and application, of religion depending on the level of consciousness of the devotee. This is also one of the reasons why in the Christian religion we have 4 Gospels that became canonical when, in fact, more than 30 exist! In simple words, there is one message for the physical, practical person-of-action, another for the emotional, romantic person, the artist, another for the intellectual and thinker, and yet another for the mystic or intuitive person.

Science "comes up from below" and works with the energies and faculties of the personality and the ego, with the *senses* (seeing and hearing in particular), with *reason,* and with one's personal *understanding* (for the social sciences use not only observation but also personal experience as their "measuring yard-sticks"). Hence it works with *human effort* and normal persons who utilize the left brain hemisphere and it operates through the male polarity. Its language is descriptive and analytical and is well defined and operationalized with one essential set of denotations which are known and accepted by those who use it. Its fundamental concepts and presuppositions are that only that which can be seen or experienced and, in some manner, *measured* and *repeated* (by those who used the same procedures), can be called "scientific".

Many other areas of reality and human experience do exist but they are defined to be outside of the pale of science. Thus science does not take the great personal and qualitative differences that exist between people into account and essentially works with the *lowest common denominator* that is available to all "normal persons" who are properly trained and who abide by the rules of science. As such it gives one practical knowledge and power which can be used, in different ways by different people, for both *good* and *evil*. The goal of science is a full realization and incarnation, the manifestation and objectification of something and not simply intuitions, thoughts, or feelings!

Going back to what I mentioned before, The Prince (science), who has arrived at a certain level of consciousness and being, will wake up the sleeping Princess (the soul or higher levels of consciousness which include the spiritual dimension) with a kiss (through love and affection). We should also now be moving from the "religion of the Son" to the "religion of the Holy Spirit"; from the personality to the soul, from the ego to the Self, and from matter to spirit; for this is what the great crisis, transition and transformation, we are now experiencing really implies. So "what comes down from above" and what "rises from below" must eventually meet . . . and this time is *now*!

One final consideration: the Great Intelligence that created us and that maintains us in existence, allowing us to go through our self-actualization and becoming, really knew what It was doing! Divine Providence is thus much wiser than human beings and their technical knowledge. This is the reason why the *knowledge and power* that we could get were always *proportional to our level of consciousness and being*; the uncreated Light and the powerful higher energies are not available to human beings until they reach a certain level and threshold . . . lest they really wreak havoc both in the world and in themselves. As we moved from our "childhood" into our "adolescence" we have greatly increased the amount of knowledge and power that is available to us . . . but how have we used this power? And how would we have used even greater powers and knowledge had they been available to us?

To be sure, there are much higher forms of knowledge and much greater powers (at the physical, psychic, and spiritual level) than the ones that we know and use. Some of these were known and used by the Saints, Sages, and Prophets (by persons who had accessed their spiritual consciousness and their soul level) who have worked "miracles" and left traces of them behind. All of these and more, we also have at the potential and latent level and we will be *able to access* as we raise our level of consciousness and as we transform this *knowledge* and *power* into *wisdom* and *love* to do God's Will, to work for the good of the whole.

And so, it is a true blessing and divine benediction that these have not been available to us until we reach a higher level of maturity. But now the time has come for us to become aware of these and to access them in that we will need them to survive and thrive in the 21st Century, to heal ourselves, our environment, and the planet! And here the fundamental axiom is very simple: true knowledge and power must always be subservient to love, to further the "good of the whole" and thus God's Will and Plan! Thus, I see a *spiritual science* which is now emerging and that will reunite both secular science and sacred religion. And it is this "spiritual science", bringing together religion and science that will develop the "new encyclopedia" and the "compendium of human knowledge" in the 21st Century!

To survive and thrive in the 21st Century, religion and science (together with the other social institutions such as health-care, education, politics, the economy, the family, etc.) will have to recognize and integrate the *spiritual dimension* which must now, because of the level of consciousness and evolution we have reached, be added to the biophysical, psychosocial, and sociocultural one. There simply is no other way! When this will occur (and it will probably occur in an "organic fashion" over a fairly long period of time) then we will witness and participate in a tremendous Renaissance and renewal of religion, of science, and of all the other social institutions as well as of the individual who will then have a far more conscious, meaningful, purposeful and enjoyable life—who will be able to live Life as it was meant to be lived, without fear or guilt, and with great zest, joy, and appreciation.

Wars, illnesses, depression, isolation, jealousy, anger, frustration, egoism, hedonism, reductionism, materialism, etc. will slowly diminish and become things of the past! For then, we shall enter the "Promised Land", the new "heaven" (level of consciousness) and the new "earth" (sociocultural world), foreseen and promised by all religions, because having reached a higher level of consciousness and being we shall create, through our knowledge, love, and will, inspired and guided by God, this "Promised Land"! The essential characteristics of the "religion of the Holy Spirit": the union of science and religion, of knowledge and intuition, love and power, of human effort and grace, and of the male and female polarities, are then likely to be the following:

1. It will have to be truly *universal* (as science always aimed and claimed to be) and cease to be *tribal* (for some but not others as most religions still are). It will teach and put into practice the fact that we all come from the same Source to return to that Source and thus that are all related and connected to each other, that we are, indeed, brothers and sisters!

2. That at the highest level we are indeed ONE, part of the same mystical body and that thus what we do unto others we ultimately do unto ourselves. Not only, but that the best way to obtain and keep something is to make it available to others, give it to others!

3. It will have to be based on a sound *physics* and *metaphysics* (which are in consonance with our present level of consciousness and being). Thus, it will have to provide and illustrate an integral theory of human nature and a holistic model of the psyche, showing that a human being is, indeed, "created in the image of God", i.e. a microcosm of the macrocosm and the point of intersection for all dimensions of reality.

4. That a human being is essentially, an *immortal spiritual being*, who has a very long past and an even longer future; who has lost the consciousness and memory of his immortality (with the Fall) which he will be able to regain them (with the Resurrection). That he is a *multidimensional* being who lives in a *multidimensional* world and that he can become aware of these higher dimensions and integrate them with the lower ones. Thus, that he will come back to the earth as many times as it is necessary for him to learn all of its lessons and actualize all of his potentialities. That there is a law of cause and effect, action and reaction such that "he

will reap what he sowed" and that what he does to others, in the end he does it to himself . . . and which is known as the law of Karma in the East. It is these two laws (reincarnation and karma) that ensure *divine justice* and the *actualization of our enormous potentials* thus giving us a sense of hope and justice in the realization that there are no "privileged or lucky persons" and that no honest effort and sacrifice will ever be in vain.

5. It will also have to develop a genuine science of grace and the sacraments which include the 7 energy-bodies, the Tree of Life with its 10 Spheres or psychospiritual centers; the law of *resonance* and *consonance* such that "only like can know like"; and that the key to genuine wisdom, love, and life or power is *wholeness* or *holiness* rather than intellectual knowledge or techniques and hi-tech gadgets! Finally, as Reality is One and composed of energies and vibrations with certain frequencies, any part of that Reality is always connected with all the others parts and can "communicate" with them by "tuning in" to their specific frequency.

6. It will have to be explain, show and demonstrate how the Christian ritual and sacramental system are connected with our energy-bodies and our psychospiritual centers, what they activate and make available to us as well as how to utilize the wonderful opportunities and potentials that they make available. How they establish certain connections and make certain energies and vibrations available . . . provided we utilize them and draw upon them!

7. That salvation can only be *collective* and global, never *individual* and thus that we are all important, need each other, and must learn to love and help each other . . . if we wish to really help ourselves. In other words, that the most important principle for our own growth and evolution, for that actualization of our latent faculties and potentialities, is *human interaction*, the law of exchange or to give to and receive from with others and the *expression of love*.

8. It will emphasize and teach the threefold process of *forgiveness* which is truly essential. Being incomplete beings who are still undergoing and evolution, we cannot avoid making mistakes just as others cannot avoid them. Hence, to learn how to forgive ourselves and others will truly is essential. This, incidentally, is a threefold process which involves *human effort* (at the mental, cognitive, and behavioral level, and which depends on us) and *divine grace* (at the emotional level and which does not depend on us).

9. It will have to recognize and act upon the fact that human beings need to be *helped* not *judged* and *condemned* and that *higher*, spiritual, *help* is *absolutely essential* at this historical juncture. Recognizing the fact that

we will not make it into the next major phase of our evolution unless we have grace, *Light*: higher energies, laws, and levels of consciousness, it will facilitate the awakening and training of these higher, spiritual principles through the example and guidance of those who have already achieved them to a certain extent.

10. It will have to redefine "sin" or human weaknesses as involving essentially "not being true to ourselves and to our destiny", and not accomplishing what we came in this world to do rather than moral or ethical principles. It will also have to teach and make quite clear that all "*sins*" will be forgiven by God (as we learn to forgive ourselves and others) *except one* (known to the Christian religion as the "sin against the Holy Spirit"). The one "mistake" that will not and cannot be forgiven is the one whereby a person *gives up on Life*, falls prey to despair, feels that there is no hope, and thus makes no effort to learn, to "get up when he has fallen", and simply "shuts down" and seeks to "escape reality" instead of learning how to cope with it!

11. It will have to provide a proper understanding of the nature, functions, dynamics and contributions of *symbolic and analogical language* so that people will be able to "work with" and "make come alive" the Sacred Scriptures and prayers of humanity which will then, by degrees, reveal to them their mysteries and treasures.

12. Last but not least, it will have to develop and incarnate a *theory and practice of love* (my term for that is the "love vitamin theory"), showing what love is, why it is so important, and how we can cultivate it and manifest it in our own lives and being.

Obviously more points could be added and probably will be added as this "spiritual science" and "religion of the Holy Spirit" emerge, unfold, and manifest themselves. But the above could be seen as a good platform and "starting point". Life on earth is going to becoming more difficult, more demanding, and more stressful, so we will really have to focus on what is *truly essential* to survive the present period and pass our *evolutionary exam*. Thus, it will be fundamental that religion, science and all the other social institutions really provide *concrete information and help* that will make a difference in people's life. This will require, above all, genuine **altruistic love**, but it will also require knowledge and wisdom, will power, courage and life!

In the West, the spiritual tradition that is rooted in the Egyptian religion and manifested through the Jewish, Christian and Moslem faiths have always prophesized and taught that the Chosen One would come to redeem fallen humanity, re-establish a living and conscious connection with God, and bring forth the Kingdom of God on earth: peace, brotherhood, health, love, and true happiness. Interestingly enough, they all point to the same *essential truth* expressed in different words and which can be interpreted in different ways on different levels of consciousness and being. Thus, the Jews are still waiting for the Messiah to come to Earth, the Christian expect the Second Coming of Christ, and the Moslem, the arrival of the Imam Madhi! They expect Him to come in the world and to set right all the human problems.

From a spiritual viewpoint, the Chosen One, the Christ, has come and has given us the archetype and prototype of what we can and must become, and He has brought the "owner's manual" by which we can live and enflesh the life that will make this possible, the Gospel of Love, Compassion, Charity, Grace and Faith. What has yet to happen and which, I believe, might well happen in the 21st Century is the *concrete realization of this in the world*. The essential "explanatory key" to understand and then realize this is very simple and logical: The Christ must now *come back in the heart, soul, and consciousness of **every human being**, and that means YOU . . . and not just One Person in the world! Thus it will be an "inner, personal, and psychic event" rather than an "external, historical and material event".

The early Christian truly believed that Jesus would come back very soon, before "this generation shall pass away" as He, Himself, had promised. And this is precisely what has happened! In every generation, He is born as a "baby", who has to grow and reach maturity, in the heart, soul, and consciousness of the few who have prepared for such event. This is what will constitute the true "salvation", of the individual and of humanity, when each person will have reached spiritual "adulthood" and "maturity", when the creature will invite the Creator, after having prepared and "adequate vehicle" of manifestation for Him. And then man will become the Man-God and will have achieved his purpose on earth.

For this Great Work, the union of human effort and grace, of the male and female polarity, of the inner and the outer dimensions, are necessary for the Man-God to be born. Perhaps, the most important "key" and insight for the full participation and realization of this is that whatever we sought in the *outer dimension*, in the world, history and others, we must now seek in the *inner dimension*, within our own being and consciousness! This is the great "secret" of the Saints and Sages and of all genuine Mystics: "When I find You, I find myself and when I find myself I find You!" It also constitutes the basic distinction between the *exoteric* and the *esoteric* aspect of religion that we find in all religions and spiritual traditions and why, in the 21st Century, they must be reunited!

Even though we cannot complete this work by ourselves and need God to complete it within ourselves, **no one** can do this for us. All human beings (and this means *you and I*) must grow up, evolve, use their free will and complete the preparatory work! And this is also what the "new encyclopedia", or compendium of all human knowledge will be all about. It will also bring together *human effort* (reason, observation, and experience) and *divine grace* (intuition, inspiration, revelation) . . . and no one can really do it fully for you because you will have to complete it and live it for and by yourself!

Conclusion and synopsis

In the second part of this work, "Religion and Spirituality", I have sought to move beyond the "body" of religion, of the various ideologies and philosophies proposed by the various religions to their very core and substance, namely to the "end" that the means are designed to achieve—authentic and *living spirituality*. For let us not forget that religions are always the means and never the end (lest they turn into "idols" which, they, themselves, warn us about!). It is most difficult to do so in cognitive, rational terms, in that by definition spirituality can only be *unique personally lived experiences* which, however, turns out to be very similar, if not identical, when people reach the same level of consciousness, being, and experience in the world. Strangely enough, we can say, at this level, that what is most *unique and personal*, at the higher levels, also turns out to be also most *universal*, perhaps because the ultimate Reality is One just as we are One at the highest levels!

After a brief exploratory journey into the major living religions of the world, what characterizes them, what they have in common and how they differ from each other, we attempted to have a look at what lies behind the great world religions, their symbolism, archetypes, and myth—their "body"; at the fundamental set of assumptions and presuppositions that constitute the bedrock of the spiritual tradition so as to penetrate into their "soul". And what is their "soul" if not the set of meanings, implications and applications, of associations and correspondences, of their *symbolism*, that we can find within the microcosm and apply to our own consciousness and being. If it is, indeed true, that there is an evolution and a destination for both man and the universe, then as we change, as our consciousness grows and unfolds, these meanings and correspondences must also change. As for the "spirit" of religion, this is something that only *personal experience* and *silence* can describe. We could describe some of the *empirical manifestations* of the "spirit" of religion but not the reality or *noumena* behind them.

The essential "explanatory" keys, or "decoding program", of spirituality is quite simple. It consists in the trinity of applying the microcosm/macrocosm analogy or relating all the symbols, archetypes, myths and their *personae dramatis* and *events* to human nature, to *ourselves* in the here and now. This is made possible by the proper understanding and application of *symbolic* and *analogical language* with its various levels and layers of interpretation which are a function of our level of consciousness and being. Obviously, this entails a great deal of personal work, of commitment and motivation, of patience and endurance, so that we can reach the higher levels of consciousness where the intuition and inspiration can flow freely . . . and unveil the mysteries and treasures of the symbols we are working with. Naturally, these two fundamental elements must culminate in a *direct and growing personal experience* of the candidate, modulated by his present level of consciousness and being, which only *silence* can properly express.

We have seen that the 21st Century will be the century of the awakening of spiritual consciousness and of the development of a spiritual science that will "wake up the sleeping Princess", namely our soul. At this point, we really no longer have a choice for, as we passed from childhood into adolescence, we are beginning to awake and harness some of the powers and potentialities of the mind and the will which, unless they are guided by a higher perspective, would greatly increase chaos, confusion, destruction and misery both in the world and in ourselves. Thus, our growth and evolution must go on and lead to into early adulthood and adulthood wherein genuine spirituality and spiritual consciousness are a *sine qua non*.

In the second part of this work, we have sought to apply the analogy of the microcosm/macrocosm and symbolic and analogical language to the Church, or temple, which is really a blue-print of ourselves—of our spiritual anatomy and physiology. Then we also applied them to two of the most important celebrations and archetypes of Christianity, Christmas and Easter; we discussed "grace" or spiritual energy, quintessential Christianity; and we ended with laying the axiological and descriptive foundation for developing a "new encyclopedia", a "compendium of human knowledge" for the 21st Century that recognizes and integrates the spiritual dimension and the spiritual tradition. To what personal experiences this work will lead you to is something that only you will be able to find out and thus to know; it will also depend largely upon your own level of consciousness and being and how much work and dedication you give to this work. But, unquestionably, something will happen as it happened with me in my youth and later in my life.

In ultimate analysis, I am also convinced that one's thought, theories, and intellectual system really are a reflection upon and a projection of one's own lived experiences and realizations—of one's *autobiography* as it were. So let me conclude the second part of the work by describing and reflecting upon some of my own personal experiences and conclusions which provide the background and foundation for the ideas, insights, and perspective which I have presented therein. As a very young child (when I was about 3 to 6 years of age), I functioned simultaneously in two very different "worlds" or dimensions: the physical one wherein most people find themselves and function in and the spiritual one, the spiritual worlds to which few people have access. Thus, I knew by direct personal experience that the spiritual worlds do exist . . . even though I could not understand what they really meant or why I had such experiences . . . which created no few problems of me at the psychological and social level.

At the age of 15, over a period of about two months, I discovered my "destiny" or what I had come to in this world, not in detail but in its essential outline. Thus, I could focus upon and give my very best to "doing my duty" and "realizing my destiny" as I clearly knew that my happiness and well-being very much depended upon this. At the age of 23, I had a major motorcycle accident that left me crippled; the best medical authorities of three countries certified that I would remain crippled for the rest of my life and that a "normal life" would, henceforth, be impossible for me. Interestingly enough, This accident and its consequences were not revealed to me at the age of 15, when I became aware of what I came to do in this world, as this would have greatly altered the way in which I lived and reacted to that truly crucial event, and prevented me from learning what I had to learn from them!

At that time, I did not believe that I could heal and have a normal life—which was essential for me to realize my destiny—and thus my life and psychological state of being were really thrown into confusion, suffering and chaos. But I still believed that "nothing happens by chance" and that there must be a very "deep and important reason" why I had the accident which I now sought to uncover and understand. To do this, I committed to and used *prayer* as the basic means to transform and expand my consciousness. Later, I completely "turned around" my way of perceiving and defining this accident from seeing it as the "worst thing that could possibly happen", to me or anyone else, to one of the "greatest gifts of God" or my true "Postgraduate School" to understand and live authentic spirituality. With a progressive understanding and acceptance of why my accident occurred also came progressive healing . . . which took at least a couple of years to complete itself.

During that time, roughly from the age of 25 to 27, I had a very difficult life, both at the physical and at the psychological level. For quite a while, I really had no idea as to what was happening to me, why it was happening, and where it would lead me to; whether it was a temporary improvement or a definitive healing. I also still experienced a great deal of pain, of fatigue, and confusion. Thus, I really needed all the help I could get and thus set upon to utilize *all the inner and outer resources* that were available to me. My family was quite comfortable at the socioeconomic level and I had a wide range of options opened to me in several countries. As I knew that it was part of my destiny that I come and live in the USA, I decided to return to New York as soon as possible and to complete my studies there.

Cognitively and practically, psychologically and physically, I was quite weak, confused, and bewildered and found it very difficult to, once again, function on my own and continue my studies even though at a lower pace than for most students. As I had already traveled in many countries, met Saints and Sages, encountered genuine healers, and studied at a very prestigious American university, culturally and educationally, I had a wide panoply of choices opened to me. I considered psychology, psychotherapy, philosophy, religion and literature as well as spiritual and esoteric schools. What I was really looking for and needed were two essential things: First a *proper perspective*, or theoretical framework, to explain what was happening to me and what I was living through—I needed greater *meaning* and *understanding*. Second, I needed the proper "instruments" to provide *hope* for my mind, *motivation* for my heart, and *energy* for my will to keep me going.

I really did not care as to where, from what discipline and through what persons, this "perspective": and "instruments" would come from. What I was essentially concerned with was that they would *work* and truly *help* me for, without help, I was convinced, several times, that I would not be able to make it and to keep on going! Thus, I had to move beyond ideology, philosophy, and consensual validation to something that was simple, natural, inexpensive, and truly effective, yielding results that I could feel and that would make an immediate difference in my life—that would enable me to keep going even when this seemed impossible from a rational viewpoint. Even before my motorcycle accident, I knew about the microcosm/macrocosm analogy, about the nature and dynamics of symbolic and analogical language, and about some of the possibilities of prayer but, of course, I had not used them beyond an intellectual grasp of what they could offer.

Having returned to the United States and gone back to my studies at Columbia University, albeit at a slower than normal pace, I had the perfect opportunity and decided to take my life and present situation as the "living laboratory" to test out these possibilities. I had also found a spiritual school in New York where I could further my understanding of the "esoteric side" of religion, in general, and of Christianity in particular. Thus, most days and on Saturdays in particular, I attended healing services and the Eastern Orthodox Liturgy on Sundays. It was at that point that I discovered, through my own personal experience, and that I began to realize what religion could really do for those truly in need. I learned about our energy-bodies, our aura, and the Tree of Life with its psychospiritual centers. I experimented with the Church being a blue-print of my own soul and consciousness and about the subtle energies and frequencies it could provide . . .

Little by little I developed and articulated the theoretical framework necessary to know myself as a *multidimensional being*, with a vertical axis of consciousness that would offer an *interdimensional* system of communication through which I could receive additional energy and life as well as the progressive healing for my battered body. I also learned to work with and utilize thought-forms, the creative (or destructive) power of thought and emotion. What conventional medicine could not do, prayer did: it not only healed me from my illness and restrictions but it also opened up a whole new universe of understanding and marvelous possibilities. Thus I discovered the deeper side and practical applications of prayer and what it could really do for us. It is then that I began to work upon a systematic approach to "esoteric Christianity" (later published as *Divine Light and Fire* and *Divine Light and Love* (Element books, 1992, and 1994).

This enabled me to get a much different and more "practical approach" to the great religious Holy Days, the interpretation of the Sacred Scriptures, and its symbolism and archetypes which, I am convinced, will play a fundamental role in the 21st Century. It also provided me with a direct, personal experience of the subtle energies and frequencies and what they can do for healing and for inspiration, and for obtaining deeper insights into aspects of the human condition. Finally, by degree and progressively, it led me to put together a new "compendium" of that kind of knowledge, or wisdom, that will be essential, as life becomes more complex and challenging, and to develop a philosophy and art of living that recognize and include the spiritual dimension.

Without authentic spirituality and its proper relationship to religion, I don't believe that I would ever have "made it" after my motorcycle accident and I would certainly not have been able to move in the direction of establishing a "spiritual science" that might well prove to be the foundation of the "Religion of the Holy Spirit". This new aspect of religion, that is essential for both religion and spirituality to remain vital and alive forces in the 21st Century, will also go a long ways to bringing together and reconciling religion, spirituality and science. In terms of our cognitive universe, of our health and well-being, there is no doubt that it will play an essential role in the years to come.

It is possible that what I had to experience in the early part of the second half of the 20th Century gave me a deeper comprehension and an "early start" in seeking for and organizing the kind of knowledge and instruments that will truly be essential for survival and, especially, for thriving in the 21st Century. For it is from this "model" and frame of reference that I have drawn the basic insights, axioms and ideas as well as the art of healing and living that have been discussed in the series, *Medicine and Spirituality*, whose essential aim was to systematically introduce and integrate the spiritual dimension in modern medicine; and that has motivated me and provided me with the basic axioms and insights for writing the present work, which I do consider, at least to date, to be my *Magnum Opus*. Time and your own personal experiences and results will confirm this . . . in one way or another.

PART III

Religion and Spirituality: their role for healthcare, wellness, and the holistic medicine of the future.

Introduction

Religion, science, and spirituality are truly the essential motive forces of human knowledge and human evolution. At different point in our human evolution and on different levels of consciousness and being, they have played different roles and have related to each other in different and even opposed ways. Basically, in our "childhood" it was religion that dominated, being inspired by authentic spirituality which, however, could not be lived by most people. When we entered our "adolescent" period, religion was replaced by science and science stood in opposition to both religion (which it saw as an obsolete superstition) and spirituality (which it could not understand rationally). But science, while it gave us great knowledge and powers (essentially over the outer physical world) also created great problems and challenges (which we are now all facing) and failed to bring about its great promise of progress: the peace in the world, health for the individual, and happiness and fulfillment for the greatest number.

This is something that only *genuine spirituality* can achieve by giving us the "larger, higher, and more global perspective" that is necessary for this to happen; by linking us consciously with the inexhaustible Source of Life, Love and Wisdom that already dwells in our superconscious; and by getting us to work for the "good of the whole" rather than for the "personal interests of the part"! At the present point in our evolution and given the level of consciousness and being we have achieved, we are still very much *incomplete beings* undergoing an evolution and, as such, cannot avoid making mistakes even important ones! Hence, we need patience and forgiveness, faith, courage and perseverance, and, especially, hope, motivation, and life to keep going forward, no matter how confusing and hard our lives and personal predicaments can be.

Essentially, we "conquered the world" but "lost our souls" . . . which we are now looking for! We realize that with proper study and research, reason and our senses, science and technology, we can get what the world has to offer, but even the best that it has to offer no longer seems either enough or truly fulfilling . . . so we want *other things* and do not yet know what we truly want, what will really bring the fulfillment and satisfaction that we hunger for. The so-called New Age is thus leaving the physical and psychological realm to begin exploring the *psychic realms*, which do exist and which are very complex, but that do not constitute the spiritual realm . . . with which it is too often confused!

It is only when we reach our adulthood or, more specifically what I called our 5th level (of consciousness and evolution) that of the "Sage" and later that of the "Saint", and that we have "passed our spiritual Puberty", or "awakening", that we can access that 5th level . . . where, at last, the "puzzle of our lives and identity can come together", and where the different approaches can be reconciled and put into proper perspective. It is at that level that religion, science, and spirituality, together with philosophy, literature—the social sciences and the humanities—can come together . . . in a proper perspective and in a grand synthesis!

Thus, the "fundamental questions of Life" remain with us; those of human identity, human suffering, and human destiny in general; and those of health, peace, morality, and personal well-being in particular. In fact, they may never have been as "actual, important, and hotly-debated" (with different and contradictory conclusions) as they are today. With the expansion of consciousness and the harnessing of higher and more powerful forms of energy, it seems that the quest for *meaning and significance*—for understanding rationally what we are living through—, for *health and well-being*, and for a sense of *purpose and destiny*, have never been greater.

This can now be explained in a very rational and scientific way: human consciousness is, unquestionably, a form of energy with its specific frequencies. As we raise our level of consciousness and being and tap higher forms of energy, the creative and destructive power of our thoughts and feelings greatly increase, for good or for evil—for creating or for destroying! Hence, it is becoming more important than ever to be able to focus, direct, and *express positive thoughts and feelings* and *avoid negative ones* for these create thought-forms that can greatly increase their power both at the *psychological* and at the *physical* level. Quantum physics, in fact, which studies the relationship and passage from the invisible and non-material to the visible and material level—from the wave-like phenomena to the particle ones—clearly states that it is the *attention* (will and thought) and the *intention* (desire and emotion) of the observer that can change the first into the second, that can manifest the invisible and non-material in a visible and material form!

There are certain very basic things that human beings have always, consciously or unconsciously, overtly or covertly, sought in all times and places. Briefly put, these are: self-knowledge and self-mastery, life and health, happiness and self-expression, and a sense of meaning and purpose in their complex and contradictory lives and being. In the present work, we are going to focus upon and limit ourselves to *life* and *health* which could be expressed as *well-being* and we are going to explore and analyze together what religion and spirituality might contribute to enhance our health and well-being.

Human beings are truly "homo religiosus", who aspire to perfection and eternity; thus religion and spirituality have always "been around" and must be recognized and taken into account, but they must be understood properly and be in sync with the level of consciousness and being of the person who utilizes them. For they do have very substantial and distinctive contributions to offer, particularly at the crucial and difficult period we are now living through—the "crisis of adolescence"! More than any other social institution or approach, religion and spirituality can tap higher levels of consciousness and being, entities and energies, laws and principles that can penetrate beyond the veil of appearances to the very core of reality, of human nature and human problems—to the essence of the human condition!

In the first chapter of this third part or volume of this work, we shall, focus our attention and direct our investigations to the very special period of time in which are presently living; we shall seek to "bring together", summarize and highlight all of the basic points, the core ideas and insights, that were mentioned throughout this work as well as in other works I have authored. Using the parable of the Prodigal Son, the journey of involution and evolution as well as the image of the human sky-scraper and the analogy of the vertical axis of consciousness, we shall seek to gain closure on what I called the "crisis of adolescence" with its "maturity exam", the passage from the reign of the personality to that of the soul, or rising from the stage of the "person of talent" to that of the "disciple" and integrating our personality with our individuality or soul.

This should provide us with an evolutionary and explanatory perspective of the paradoxes and contradictions, the trials and tribulations, the confusion and disorder, which now exist both in ourselves and in the society and culture we have created. It should be of great help to enable us to understand what we are presently living through by looking at and putting it into proper perspective where we are coming from and where we are going. As such, this chapter should offer a major contribution in understanding better religion, spirituality, health-care, and wellbeing, as well as their relationship to each other.

In the second chapter, I propose to do the same thing with the basic assumptions, presuppositions, the core intuitions and ideas, that were mentioned throughout this work and in other books and papers I authored, so as to give coherence and intellectual objectivity to the "new/old way" of looking at religion, spirituality, healthcare and their interrelationships. The central point here is both clear and simple: if you understand and are in agreement with these assumptions, then all the rest follows, logically and rationally, if you don't then, obviously, you will not be able to follow and profit from what is being suggested here. And, ultimately, this is a question and a reflection of your own personal and present level of consciousness and being to which you must be faithful as it is all you have to work with!

The third chapter will continue this journey and exploration by seeking to discover and highlight the specific role that religion and spirituality can play for the emerging paradigm of the medicine and health-care of the 21st Century. Rather than ignoring them or putting them in opposition to the medicine of the future, these must be faced, studied, and properly integrated so as to discover and utilize the very major contributions they can make on various levels—preventive, therapeutic, educational, and philosophical.

The fourth chapter will follow and continue logically the discourse and analysis begun in the third chapter. Specifically, it will attempt to identify and highlight the distinctive contributions that religion and spirituality can make to our health and well-being; how their theoretical perspective and the practical instruments they make available to us can significantly help us preserve our health, restore it when we have fallen prey to various pathologies, and enable us to grow—to consciously continue our evolution by raising our level of consciousness and being.

The fifth chapter will seek to complete this journey and exploration by suggesting practical ways in which religion and spirituality can be integrated both in our personal lives and being, and in our profession, the healthcare profession in particular. One of the core assumptions of the spiritual perspective is that everything is interrelated and interacting, thus that everything is important and relevant! This is particularly true of religion and spirituality which can make a very significant difference in the way we live and in the way we serve others through our selected profession.

Thus, the third part or "volume" of this work will attempt to bring together, relate, and be of theoretical and practical use for our readers, integrating the fundamental insights and ideas of the first two parts as well as of many of my other articles, essays, and books. If its fundamental assumptions, insights and ideas are correct, they should make a noticeable difference in both our personal and our professional life—they should help us know, master and express ourselves better in a world that will no longer be hostile or unintelligible but a true "laboratory" for our own growth and becoming. They should help us understand what "marvel we are" and what "incredible gift" is life on the material plane, on earth, in spite of all of its contradictions, confusion, and difficulties.

Chapter I

THE GREAT CHALLENGES OF OUR TIMES, THEIR DANGERS AND OPPORTUNITIES

As it is well-known to both the spiritual tradition and now also to the growing social sciences, if we want to truly know ourselves in an objective and comprehensive manner, we need to know and understand the environment and the historical period in which we find ourselves; to know ourselves we need to know the world in which we live because these really are two facets of the same coin! Now each historical period and its physical environment are *unique*, with their distinctive characteristics, dangers and opportunities. But, somehow, the historical juncture we find ourselves in at the end of the 20th and the beginning of the 21st Century, or more precisely the hundred years that began around 1950 and that will end around 2050, are very special and unique.

It may, in fact, turn out to be the crucial and pivotal "crossroads" of our evolution, with enormous and very real dangers but equally enormous and maybe even greater opportunities. To answer what I call the "fundamental questions of our times", it is essential that we gain a proper understanding of that historical period, that we put it into a proper perspective, and that we avoid its most important dangers and capitalize on its greatest opportunities.

For we are living not only at the end of a century and at the beginning of a new millennium, but also at a time when humanity, collectively speaking, is moving from its childhood to its adulthood through the phase that, at the individual biological level, we call "adolescence" but which can also be applied at the larger, collective and evolutionary, level. This period of time is fraught with very major quantitative and qualitative changes and transformations which imply great dangers and risks but also great opportunities and rewards, both at the individual and at the collective level. The great mystics, seers, and thinkers of our race, the great souls that we find in every race, religion and part of the world as well as some of our finest thinkers, researchers, and educators have all "sensed" this and sought to understand it and describe it to us in different languages and cultural clothing.

This historical juncture has been called the "Apocalypse", the "Kali Yuga", the "Period of great Tribulations or Purification", and even the "End of Times" by the sacred traditions of different races and religions. It has also been viewed as the "post-industrial", "information", or "globalization" age by the academic scholars and thinkers of our times, which would be responsible for great quantitative and qualitative changes that will have a profound impact on our religion, politics, employment, education, the family, and, especially, our physical and psychological health. Great political and economic polarizations would arise that would involve religious and moral wars and clashes, new illnesses, super viruses, and a tremendous amount of confusion, disorder, and stress as people would find life becoming evermore demanding and thus complex, difficult, confusing and especially stressful . . . with a major impact on both our psychological and our physical health.

On the other side of the coin, however, new horizons and possibilities will also open up for greatly expanding our knowledge, our ability to understand ourselves, the world in which we live, and the purpose for which we came into this world; for being much better able to express ourselves and create a more human, meaningful, and rewarding life. At long last, at this historical juncture, it will be possible, for an ever-increasing number of persons, to be able to answer the "riddle of the Sphinx" (who am I? Whence do I come from, whither am I going, and what have I come to do in this world?) and thus to express oneself through increased knowledge, love and creativity. It will also become possible to reconcile opposites and to explain paradoxes and contradictions at a higher level and thus make possible a true "compendium or synthesis of human knowledge" that can greatly help us complete our being and evolution, as well as create the environment and life-style that are healthy, moral, and in accordance with our destiny.

To avoid the risks and dangers of this historical period as well as to be able to profit from the opportunities and possibilities that it opens for us, it will be essential for us to raise our level of consciousness and to be able to access higher laws, principles and energies than those made available by the black box of science of the 20th Century, namely, our reason, our will, and our senses. Thus we will have to be able to access *grace*, spiritual Light or energies, and to move from the "Reign of Nature" to that of "Grace". For at the very heart and core of this massive quantitative and qualitative transformation we find the *expansion and elevation of our consciousness* which does require integrating higher energies and frequencies the nature and origin of which can only be *spiritual*!

At a simple and practical level this means that we will no longer be able to afford living as we have lived before and to indulge in the "human weaknesses and vices" which have characterized our past and which have reached their culminating point at the present time. Thus we will have to "rediscover" the traditional virtues and morality, to develop rigor and integrity, and to discipline our inner and outer lives by gradually transmuting negative thoughts, feelings, and states of mind into positive ones . . . or risk much worse diseases, sufferings, and the destruction of our physical vehicle.

This can be explained by a very simple but fundamental fact: *as we raise our level of consciousness and bring in more Life, higher energies, we also increase, in direct proportion the creative or destructive power of our thoughts, feelings, and psychological states.* This means that, more and more, we will literally *create our illnesses and sufferings* . . . or *their resolution* . . . and healing, peace, harmony, and justice in the world or war, imbalances, and destruction, which we will then have to assume and live through! In summary, we could say that our present time is characterized by the following basic trends:

- *Polarization*: having to choose and then act upon a given choice . . . where even refusing to choose becomes a choice in itself!
- *Intensification*: everything becomes more powerful and intense, for good or for evil, for life and health or illness and death, and for joy or for suffering.
- *Acceleration*: everything is now happening at a faster and faster rate. What used to take years, months, or weeks is now taking days, hours or seconds, or even happens in "real time" that is instantaneously!
- *Etherialization*: what we call "reality" or "truth" is now appearing more and more as a "conscious process" or a "psychological entity" and less and less as a material, external one.

Underlying all of this, of course, is our own psyche or the *transformation and expansion of consciousness*—moving from one floor of the inner sky-scraper to a higher one, actualizing our faculties and potentialities, or becoming *in fact* what we already are *potentially*. Signs of this are everywhere and manifest in a multitude of different and even opposed ways which, nevertheless, are very "real" and all point to the same thing: the raising of our consciousness—being able to know and understand more, to feel and experience more, and to express ourselves and create more!

At the cognitive level, the spiritual tradition has given us to very important "points of reference" . . . which we can corroborate in our own being and lives when we reach the necessary level of consciousness and being. These are: the *Parable of the Prodigal Son*, which describes our enormous journey and extraordinary adventure in the worlds of Creation, showing us where we come from, where we are going and what is the specific point of our becoming in which we now find ourselves. And the *theory of the human sky-scraper* . . . that likens a human being to a sky-scraper with multiple floors and an inner elevator that can move and down those floors.

The parable of the Prodigal Son tells us that we came from the spiritual worlds to eventually return to them; that we are all the "Prodigal Son" or "solar hero"; and that God, or the Ultimate Reality, is our "Father", or Creator and Sustainer, so that we participate in His nature and capabilities . . . to the extent that we remain "connected with Him and participate" in His Attributes, Will, and Plan. This long journey can best be represented with a "V" composed of three essential parts: the *descent into matter*, or moving away from our "essence and home", the *ascent back to spirit*, or returning to our "essence and home", and the point where our *motion inverts*, where the descent now turns into the ascent! Religion calls the first the "Fall" and the second the "Redemption". As for the third part, it is called the "Return of the Savior" preceded by the "Apocalypse".

The spiritual tradition views the first as the process of "involution", the second as the process of "evolution", and the third as the "great turning point" . . . where consciousness and culture can no longer descend further into matter and must turn back to spirit! In more modern and perhaps humoristic terms, I like to call the first the "plunge into matter and amnesia", the second the "great awakening" or discovery of our identity, and the third the "crisis of adolescence" with its "maturity exam" which is the final, culminating point, where we "touch bottom" so that can now truly "turn around" . . . and get back on the "tracks of our destiny" and the "purpose for which we were created".

While we are definitely in the period of the Apocalypse, or the "crisis of adolescence", we have not yet, at least collectively speaking, "touched bottom" and "taken our exam"! That is something which is yet to come and that will occur in the near future. When exactly it will occur and what specific aspect it will take, only God knows, as human will and freedom of choice can make a difference . . . so that the future is never fully determined or "written in cement". That moment, however, is quite close and is drawing closer every day . . . Until such time, life on earth all over the world will become evermore complex, confusing, difficult, and stressful! This means that more and more people will find it increasingly difficult to meet their obligations and to "keep going" and that many will be unable to do so and thus be confronted with either giving up on life . . . or turning to the vertical dimension and to seek grace, higher energies and inspiration!

As for the theory of the human skyscraper (which I have already discussed in greater details elsewhere), it argues, essentially, that while we are all functioning in the same material world, we do not all function on the same level of consciousness and being and thus do not perceive reality, a given situation or event, in the same way. Thus there are also 7 basic types of persons even though the last 3 are still extremely rare so that, for practical purposes, we have

4 types of persons, hence 4 different ways of perceiving and defining the reality with have to deal with. These are the "primitive person" (the baby), the "normal person" (the child), the "person of talent" (the adolescent), the "disciple" (the young adult), followed by the "Sage", the "Saint", and the "fully realized Person" (respectively, the adult, the mature adult, and the older person).

From this viewpoint or "point of reference" our present historical times represent the *passage from the "person of talent" to the "disciple" and, eventually to the "Sage"*. These different levels and ways of perceiving and defining reality can be seen, quite clearly, in religion and healthcare, which can explain their strange, confusing and paradoxical relationship to each other. Institutionalized religion in the West, by and large and regardless of its particular kind (whether Jewish, Christian, or Muslim) is still at the 2nd stage, that of the "normal person" or of the "child". Science is clearly at the 3rd level, that of the "person of talent", or that of the "adolescent", and the so-called New Age movement is at the 4th level, that of the "disciple" or that of the "young adult".

It is only at the 5th level and above, that of the "Sage" and "Saint" or of the "adult" and "mature adult", that these can be put into a *proper and larger perspective and reconciled*, with the proper guidance and inspiration from above, so that each will find its proper place, function, and characteristics. Thus those who have worked (and are working) to bring about the "united religions of the world" and a way to reconcile and integrate human knowledge and human experience will have to wait until such level is realized . . . or work with people who have already reached that level! This may not sound fair, democratic, just, or equitable but it is a reality which we have to learn to accept and learn to adapt ourselves to.

At the level of healthcare and medicine, the same basic, evolutionary paradigm also applies. Ethnic and traditional medicine (which we find in non-developed and traditional societies and cultures) is located basically at the 1st and 2nd level, that of the "baby" and the "child". Modern allopathic, or physical, medicine is clearly based on the 3rd level, that of the "person of talent", as its basic point of reference and identification is "materialistic science". Alternative, holistic, and psychosomatic medicine clearly belongs to the 4th level, that of the "disciple". Finally, spiritual medicine, the approach of the great Saints, Sages, and Healers, can only be ascribed to the 5th level and beyond (that of the "Sage", the "Saint", and the fully-actualized person"). A little thought and reflection will make this thesis quite clear and rational.

The child is passive and dependent. He needs to be told what is right and what is wrong, he needs to be taken care of by "older" more experienced persons, and to be punished when he does not obey or conform. Here things are black and white, right or wrong, with little or no "shades of grey". Thus he becomes dependent upon his parents, society, and social institutions that will "socialize and educate him" into becoming a "social being, an adult and a good citizen". The adolescent, on the other hand, rebels against his parents and rejects tradition. He wants to experiment with everything and find out for himself what is true or false, good or bad, and effective or not. Here professionals, experts, and technicians replace the elder and wiser persons that provided fundamental values, moral example and guidance for the former levels and types.

As for the young adult, he begins to realize, through his own personal experience, that "man does not live by bread alone", that one can have all of one's material needs and aspirations taken care of and still *remain unsatisfied and wanting*, and that Life is much greater than its rational representation by science and its gratification through technology. Slowly but surely, persons on that level of consciousness and being, will look for deeper, non-material things, for the hidden causes and not merely the symptoms of their problems and questions. Thus, they will discover, begin to explore and then harness, the psychological and psychic side of life with strange and unusual procedures that often confuse fact and fantasy, reality and wishful thinking, and which is known under the label of the "New Age".

As for religion and science, on the lower levels they are opposed to each other as the first "descends from above" as the second "rises from below". But if something descends and something rises along the same vertical axis, at a certain point they will meet and integrate. For me this point is **today** just as it is for the reconciliation of opposites and the famed "coincidentia oppositorum"! Thus, the historical juncture we are living in is, indeed, very difficult, demanding, and challenging, but it is also incredibly rewarding and making possible for many what in the past only occurred for extremely rare and evolved persons—the realization of our greatest dreams and ambitions . . . or of our worst fears and nightmares.

According to the spiritual tradition, we have clearly chosen to incarnate at this time and to live through the challenges of this critical period—that is our soul, before incarnating in the physical world, did so in the worlds of Light. Thus, it behooves us to truly *give it our best*, not less than what we can do but not more either! And to understand and put into a proper perspective this paradox and fundamental aspect of the male and female polarities, it is essential that we know clearly what *depends on us* (human effort) and what *does not* (divine grace), what we can and should do with our personality, developed to its highest level, and what we cannot do and must ask for help from the higher powers. It is to seek to properly understand and resolve this very important paradox and question that this book and its related seminars are presented to you!

Chapter II

ESSENTIAL PRESUPPOSITIONS, INTUITIONS, CORE INSIGHTS AND IDEAS

When doing professional academic work, it is well-known and an accepted rule that we define our central terms, clearly and explicitly, and that we state our fundamental assumptions and core ideas . . . for these will definitely determine all the rest at the logical level. It is for this reason that I want define the basic assumptions, intuitions, and the core insights and ideas that underpin religion, spirituality, healthcare and their interrelationships. These are relatively few and simple but with a very important impact as they constitute the true "axiological" layer, or foundation, for this work. Here I am going to suggest the most important ones for your consideration and reflection. To simplify things I will group them around three basic subjects: *knowledge* and *human nature*, and *religion* and *spirituality*, and *health, illness,* and *healing*. Bear in mind that these are analytical, arbitrary classifications created by the human mind for, in reality, they are all interdependent and interacting seamlessly with each other.

A. *Knowledge or epistemology*: what do we know, how we know what we know, and what do we consider valid" scientific" knowledge today?

Essentially, human knowledge is a function of the level of consciousness and being of the person who develops it. It can also be subdivided into two different but complementary types of knowledge: intellectual, conceptual knowledge about something—*knowledge ab extra*—or knowledge about something which we create mentally and intellectually; and direct experiential knowledge of something—*knowledge ab intra*—knowledge of something that we experience personally. The social sciences call the first "scientific knowledge" and the second "understanding". In the first instance, there is a *subject* that beholds or *observes* an object which is different and external to the subject while in the second instance there is a *merging* of the subject and the object so that they become, temporarily, *one*, and where the subject can render conscious what was before unconscious.

The first type of knowledge, "scientific knowledge" is located on the *horizontal axis*, it is quantitative, and assumed to be "objective", i.e. to exist independently of the observer. The second type of knowledge, instead, "understanding", is located on the *vertical axis*, it is qualitative and is assumed to exist only insofar as the subject exists. The first is what we call "rational knowledge" that comes from the head while the second is "experiential and intuitive knowledge" that comes from the heart. In classical literature, the first was called "l'esprit de géométrie" and the second "l'esprit de finesse" (Blaise Pascal).

In summary and in conclusion: there are two basic types of knowledge, which complement each other, but which are quite different in their nature, origins, and expressions: cognitive, rational or *intellectual knowledge*, which our minds give us about our experiences and the objects of our environment, and *experiential, intuitive knowledge* which are hearts give us through our ability of empathy and sympathy—of uniting with our chosen subject and of rendering it conscious. The first is based on the *horizontal axis* and is quantitative, coming from our personality and enabling us to understand and survive in the physical world. The second is based on the *vertical axis* and is qualitative, coming from our soul and our spiritual Self, and enabling us to obtain meaning, purpose, and value of what lies beyond the realm of phenomena. The first is relative and limited and deals essentially with the physical, sensate world while the second is absolute and unlimited as it deals with spiritual things. The first comes from human effort, discipline and study while the second from grace, sensitivity and the principle of resonance. For our purposes, it is very important to be able to distinguish between these two forms of knowledge, to cultivate both and to be able to integrate them in our consciousness and lives.

B. *Human nature*: Who and what are we? Where do we come from? Where are we going? And why were we born in this world? What is the range of human behavior? What can we do and what can we not do?

For most people and all of the academic disciplines, at this particular point in human evolution, human nature, its origins, destiny, and capabilities are still "opaque" and partial and hotly debated by various hypotheses and theories which are different and even contradictory in nature. It is only through the awakening of spiritual consciousness and the teachings of the spiritual tradition that we can put these into a larger, more unifying perspective and understand their higher aspects and facets. More than ever, one's "theory of human nature", or vision of what man is and what man can do, is a function of the level of consciousness and being of the person involved. Structurally, however, there are three fundamental possibilities, presuppositions, or theories which have very different and important consequences. These are:

1. *Homo simplex*: Man is essentially his biological organism and consciousness is merely and epiphenomenon of biochemical processes. Thus, human nature has one basic dimension, the physical one; he comes from nothing (before birth) to return to nothing (after death) as there cannot be any consciousness, identity or will without a material base. This conception corresponds to that of the "primitive person", the baby, and is slowly disappearing at the present time. It was, however, the basic underpinning for the materialistic and rationalistic theories.

2. *Homo duplex*: Man is dual, his has a biological organism but also a psyche which can become a causal and creative agent once it developed. Human nature has two basic dimensions, the physical and the psychological. Before birth there is nothing but when a human being is conceived biologically and interacts humanly the potential for human consciousness and identity is actualized and becomes the unique and distinctive characteristic of a human being. This consciousness and identity may or may not survive the death of his biological organism. This hypothesis provided the underpinning for the psychosocial theories of the social sciences . . . until the end of the 20th Century.

3. *Homo triplex*: Man has a triple nature composed of a biopsychic organism (the body), a psychosocial entity (the psyche) and a spiritual nature (the soul and spiritual Self). While his spiritual nature constitutes the essence and mainspring of his being, it remain unconscious for a long period of time, until a person reaches his "spiritual puberty", wakes up his spiritual consciousness, and brings it unto consciousness, control and integration. This is the central thesis of the spiritual tradition and of all spiritually-oriented thinking.

A human being is thus a *multidimensional* being, who is still undergoing a long evolution and is composed of at least three basic natures and dimensions, the physical (biopsychic), the human (psychosocial) and the spiritual (psychospiritual). He is truly a microcosm of the macrocosm and the point of intersection of all dimensions and aspects of reality. His fundamental evolutionary goal is to awaken his consciousness, become self conscious, and enable both nature (Spirit's immanent aspect) and God (Spirit's transcendent aspect) to become conscious. In order to perceive, interact, and make exchanges with something outside of himself, man must first awaken the *corresponding part within himself*. Thus, to function in the physical world, he needs a physical body;

to function in the psychic worlds he needs energy-bodies, and to function in the spiritual world, he needs a spiritual body . . . as "only like can know like"!

The growth and unfoldment of his consciousness follows directly the growth and unfoldment of his being. It involves a very long evolutionary journey and countless experiences to translate potentiality into actuality. The central process by which consciousness develops and faculties are actualized is *interaction*, the give and take, with something outside of himself. It follows the same line of development of his being which is such that first he develops physical awareness with the perfection and utilization of his physical body; then comes human consciousness with the perfection and utilization of his psyche; and finally emerges spiritual consciousness with the integration of his soul and spiritual Self with his psyche which can then manifest them.

At the present stage, collectively speaking, a human being stands between childhood and adulthood and his going through his "crisis of adolescence" with its culminating point, the "maturity exam". This implies a major transformation and expansion of consciousness that will bring psychosocial consciousness to integrate psychospiritual consciousness . . . with the birth of spiritual consciousness and the integration of his personality with his soul. This, as we have seen in the previous chapter, will bring about a major redefinition of knowledge and all of its objects as well as a new culture and life-style.

C. *Religion and Spirituality*: their basic nature and distinctive features.

Religion means to unite or to "bring together" . . . first the different natures and components of human nature and then human nature and what exists in the world: other human beings, nature and God. Religion has always existed and will always exist in this world . . . until such time as man will have actualized all of his faculties and potentialities, and realized his destiny in this world. Thus every person is, fundamentally, a *homo religiosus*, a religious being who is driven by a fundamental impulse to reach his perfection, to accomplish his destiny, to actualize all of his faculties and potentialities. The same *telos* or *élan vital* that we find in all living things, we also find in human beings but raised to a higher level and involving the full development of human consciousness.

The founders of all authentic religions, spiritual and metaphysical schools, were unquestionably *older souls* or more evolved persons who were inspired by God, divine grace, or spiritual energy. By and large they did not write books or create religions but spoke, taught, and lived certain fundamental truths and principles that can serve as "models", "guidelines", and "inspiration" to guide, direct, and accelerate our own evolution. The basic problem that arose here is that everything, religion included, must be brought down to the level of consciousness and being of the person that will teach it and live it . . . and the followers of these great Beings were, obviously on lower and different levels than the Founders of religion. Thus, the symbols, archetypes, rites and myths of religion were "translated", "codified" and "institutionalized" on lower levels of consciousness and being to touch and be meaningful to those who functioned on those levels . . . even though, when properly interpreted, they contain treasures and messages for all 7 levels of consciousness and being!

As there exist 7 basic levels of consciousness and types of persons who exemplify them, so there can be 7 different interpretations of the symbols, images, rites, and teachings of all religions. However, as the three higher ones are still extremely rare, at the practical level, we have 4 basic levels and types which can be found in the 4 Gospels of the Christian tradition. These are what I call the "primitive person" (the baby), the "normal person" (the child), the "person of talent" (the adolescent) and the "disciple" (the young adult). Beyond these, we find the "Sage" (the adult), the "Saint" (the mature adult) and the "fully actualized Person" (the elder). The dilemma and paradox or religion is that we find major clashes and antinomies between the second, the third, and the fourth level . . . that can only be reconciled and properly integrated at the *fifth level*, that of the "Sage"! As for healthcare and medicine, we find the same paradoxes and clashes but which are now focused on the third level (allopathy) vs. the fourth level (psychosomatic and alternative medicine) vs. the fifth level (spiritual medicine) and that will be recognized properly, integrated and utilized in a wise an effective fashion at the fifth level.

As for spirituality, in an authentic and lived way, it can only begin at the *fourth level* and really come unto its own and articulate a proper perspective and presentation at the *fifth level* . . . as it must be anchored in the *direct personal experience* of the devotee which begins at those levels. With the birth of spiritual consciousness and the introduction and integration of the spiritual dimension, a major transformation or paradigm shift occurs . . . which brings about a "new creature", a new identity and form of knowledge and not simply a different philosophy, ideology or theory.

Strangely enough, it could be said that "true life on earth", that is a conscious, responsible, autonomous, creative and full life really *begins with the dawning of spiritual consciousness* as it is only then that a person can truly "open its arms to life" and accept all of its experiences, paradoxes, and confusion without fear, insecurity, anguish, guilt, frustration, and rejection. As very few people have reached that "spiritual puberty" yet, we could truly say that very few people are truly "living" and that they most only "exist" . . . at the personality level which is a "shadow" level!

The spiritual dimension, which is as yet invisible and non-material, is truly the source and matrix of all there is; thus the psychic and physical dimensions are truly a manifestation or projection of the spiritual dimension which is the truly *causal dimension* where everything begins . . . and ends. The seven great planes of creation as well as the seven basic levels of consciousness and being are thus *emanations* of the spiritual dimension where the frequencies and energies are condensed, diminished, and "crystallized". Spiritual consciousness, on the other hand, could be defined as "all those levels of consciousness that lie above and beyond sensory, emotional, and mental consciousness and which underpin them".

Ultimately, spiritual consciousness cannot be defined rationally and must be *felt and experienced* as we have no adequate vocabulary to describe many of its characteristics and processes and as intellectual and cognitive definitions miss out many of its subtle nuances and aspects. Moreover, while there are many religions there is, ultimately, but *one genuine spirituality* which is "polarized" into its opposed but complementary traditions of East and West, of Being and Love, where individual consciousness fuses and "loses" itself in cosmic consciousness or where it needs a Partner to generate and manifest Love. We could also say that "religion is the means" while "spirituality" is the "end". Spiritual consciousness does however; present certain basic characteristics which are the following:

1. It will reveal and manifest, for the first time, the true identity of "Reality", both inner and outer, of our true Self and of God. Thus, it is only when we reach that level and awaken spiritual consciousness that we will, at long last, be able to answer the Riddle of the Sphinx . . . in a meaningful and lasting way: Who am I? Where do I come from? Where am I going? Why have I incarnated in this world? What should I do here and what constitutes true value and meaningful experience?

2. It will definitely and forever eliminate our greatest and most archaic source of fear, anxiety and insecurity: that of death and dying. For then we shall experience and integrate the fact that we are immortal beings, that birth and death are merely qualitative "passages" from one dimension into another and that Life is without beginning and without ending in an ascending scale of progression.

3. This, in turn, will make available a great deal more energy and vitality which we will be able to use through our three "ontological qualities" of knowing and understanding, of loving and feeling, and of willing and creating. On the one hand, it will free a great deal of psychic energy that before was "dissipated" or burnt up in fears, anxieties, frustrations, and negative thoughts and feelings. On the other hand, it will also make accessible spiritual energies, which are related but distinct from psychic and physical energies. And this will truly make our lives "more abundant"!

4. It will lead us to what the French call "la joie de vivre", the joy of being alive—the ability to accept, appreciate and be grateful for all that we live and experience as we realize that its is meaningful, that it does

"lead somewhere" and that it will enrich us and enable us to become more than what we are.

5. It will also give us the "keys" to *true knowledge* (of ourselves, of God and of Nature and of their interrelations); of *true love* (of ourselves, of God, of Nature, and of others), and of *true creativity* or self-expression!

Again, bear in mind that spiritual consciousness must be realized and experienced to be truly understood as we lack the vocabulary to describe its nature, characteristics and manifestations and as these, in any case, involve a great deal more that mere "cognition" and intellectual knowledge (for example emotional experiences, creative realizations, and *sui generis* traits). Of one thing (that comes in three steps) I am truly convinced and that is: that it is our destiny to awaken and integrate spiritual consciousness with our physical and human consciousness, that this is the step major qualitative step in our evolution, and that the time for doing so is *now*!

D. *Health, Illness, and Healing*: their basic nature, dynamics and manifestations.

As you might surmise, these core concepts are also functions of our level of consciousness and evolution and change as we grow and raise our consciousness. Thus, at different stages and for different people, these may be quite different and, in any case, dynamic, emergent and evolving. Let us begin with health. What is "health": what are its basic nature, characteristics and manifestations? For a long time, health was defined simply as being the absence of disease, namely of painful and dysfunctional symptoms such as infection, inflammation, fever, swelling, pain, and weakness. The goal of healthcare was thus to identify and get rid of these dysfunctional symptoms. This view then changed to include the notion of equilibrium or "homeostasis" within the physical body which consisted of many different organs and systems that had to function in harmony with each other.

The next stage was characterized by a relentless "war" against microbes, viruses, and pathogenic elements that attacked the body as a nation can be attacked by other nations. Thus, for allopathy, it was the "war model" that was applied and used with a direct analogy between war in the world (between nations) and war within our bodies . . . where the fundamental objective was to develop evermore powerful weapons that would enable us to conquer these pathogenic agents and rid our biological organism from them. Here science and technology came to the rescue with an ever-increasing panoply of hi-tech gadgets and evermore sophisticated pharmacopoeia. Some results, at times even spectacular results were achieved. But all was not well with this approach and two major obstacles began appearing and growing on the horizon which, in the long run, will bring the demise or strong modification of this approach: it became ever-more *dangerous* and it became ever-more *expensive*!

The next qualitative breakthrough was the appearance of psychosomatic medicine and the re-evaluation of the traditional, alternative, more energy and frequency based approaches we call "holistic", unconventional or "soft". It is here that Claude Bernard finally got his vindication over Louis Pasteur and that we began to realize that, indeed, the only thing that can heal us is what the ancients called the *Vis Medicatrix Naturae* (i.e. our immune, hormonal, nervous, and circulatory systems); and so that, indeed, the microbe is nothing and the "soil" is everything. More and more people began to realize that those who live the longest and are the healthiest are not necessarily those who live in developed, rich, and industrialized countries (and who, therefore, have a modern healthcare system at their disposal) but rather those who remain close to nature, in harmony with the laws of God, and who seek to do their "duty" or fulfill their destiny!

Not too long ago, it was realized that "the greatest medical discovery of the 20th century is neither penicillin nor heart-transplants but rather the realization that "our bodies and psyches were so designed by the Creator that they can heal themselves from all known and unknown diseases . . . provided that they have the proper matter (food—nutrition) and energy (attitude, faith-psychotherapy)". To this I would personally add *destiny* as the third crucial factor in line with the teachings of the spiritual tradition. Essentially, what happened here is that, with the growth and expansion of our consciousness, we began to realize that we are, indeed, highly complex multidimensional beings who have a biological organism ruled by biochemistry . . . but that this body might only be a "symptom" or "effect" of causes and matrixes that lie on a higher qualitative level.

We began to discover that our thoughts and emotions have a powerful effect on our health, illnesses, and healing, and thus that so do our psychosocial relationships and our sociocultural environment. We began to "rediscover" the fact that we have not only a physical body but also "energy-bodies" (specifically an etheric-vital, astral-emotional, mental and spiritual body) with their own distinctive "organs" or psychospiritual centers. We also began to realize that everything is interconnected and interacting with everything else so that nothing is unimportant or should be left out; that our *vitality* or energy level plays a truly fundamental role in maintaining or restoring our health.

This brought about the realization that our thoughts and emotions, our "state of being", become increasingly more important as we raise our level of consciousness; that our main objective should be to work towards a state of *bio-psycho-spiritual harmony* wherein every cell, organ, system and, ultimately, also our ego and personality, can "fulfill their natural function". And this brought about what I call the 5th level of medicine or "spiritual medicine", which is that of the Sages, the Saints, and the genuine Healers who, with their presence, radiations, and words can restore full health and this, at times, even "at a distance" while not being present!

In synthesis, the ethnic and traditional healing approaches of primitive and traditional societies constitute the 1st and 2nd level of medicine, allopathy the 3rd level, psychosomatic and alternative medicine the 4th level and "spiritual medicine" the 5th level. These, in turn, are correlated with what I call the "primitive person" (the baby) and the "normal person (the child)—the 1st and 2nd level; with the "person of talent" (the adolescent)—the 3rd level; with the "disciple" (the young adult)—the 4th level; and with the "Sage, the Saint, the fully actualized Person" (the adult, the mature adult, and the older person)—the 5th level and beyond.

Until we cognitively reach the 5th level and are inspired by grace to see the whole structural and evolutionary picture, each level or approach is based upon certain premises that, taken by themselves, render the previous and the next one unintelligible and thus "quackery" or fantasy. Hence, it is only at the 5th level of consciousness and being that we will be able to "reconcile opposites", deal with the "coincidentia oppositorum", and be able to resolve and integrate paradoxes and contradictions into a higher perspective and synthesis that will foster genuine understanding, compassion, and proper usage of all theories and approaches.

Given the foregoing as a background and perspective, what are health, disease, and healing and their basic processes and characteristics for us today?

- *Health*: manifests itself on the four major levels of consciousness and being that make up human nature, the physical-vital, the emotional-astral, the mental, and the spiritual. On the physical-etheric level it is essentially strength, proper coordination, and vitality which enable us to use our physical bodies as a cooperative and effective instrument. On the emotional-astral level it is courage, appreciation, and gratitude—the desire to live and to experience whatever life will throw at us. On the mental level, it implies clarity and comprehension, the apprehension of cause and effect, meaning and purpose, in whatever we are living through. Finally, on the spiritual level, it implies remaining properly connected with our divine spark, the inexhaustible Source of Life, Love, and Wisdom which dwells in the depths of our being and in the heights of our consciousness.

    Health, therefore, is more than the absence of painful and dysfunctional symptoms; it is more than proper equilibrium or "homeostasis" between our various biological organs and systems; and it also is more than the sound functioning of our immune, hormonal, nervous, and circulatory systems. Health also implies growing, evolving, actualizing our faculties and potentialities; it involves the proper circulation of light, energy, and materials in our various systems and subsystems, the proper communication between our various energy-bodies and their psychospiritual centers; and it implies remaining "connected" with the Great Chain of Being and with God's Will and grace or Light.

Health, therefore, means the proper harmony, connection, and communication between our physical, our human, and our spiritual nature in the microcosm and with the physical, psychic and spiritual dimensions in the macrocosm. Thus, it is also synonymous with "peace", "justice", "harmony"—the ability to maintain the proper proportion, measure, distance and timing—so that we can fulfill God's Plan and our destiny . . . or, at least, this is as much, as can be said in words at the present time and which, in any case, will have to be lived and experienced to be properly understood.

- *Disease or pathology*: obviously implies a "break" disharmony" or temporary interruption of the foregoing. Interestingly enough, when considering illnesses and pathologies, we are confronted with a major paradox which is directly linked with the paradox of evil as illness is an aspect or facet of "evil": at the ontological level, *sub species aeternitatis*, disease and evil do not exist, only health and good exist in that there only God exist! It is at the existential level, *sub species temporalis*, that disease and evil exist . . . but on a temporary and not a permanent basis! While good, life and health have no beginning and no end as they are "real" and exist forever; whereas evil and disease always have a beginning and an end as they only "exist" on the four lower planes of creation! Hence, we could say that they are temporary "disharmonies", "imbalances", blockages" that need to be "readjusted" or harmonized and removed.

  On the physical plane, illness manifests as weakness, lack or coordination, pain, infection, inflammation, etc. whereby we can no longer use our bodies as an efficient instrument. On the emotional plane, it manifests as fear, anxiety, insecurity, anguish, guilt, frustration, hatred—the whole panoply of negative emotions and feelings that have a feed-back loop with both our physical and our psychological nature. On the mental plane, it implies confusion, misunderstanding, the inability to perceive causal relationships and meaning, purpose and value in whatever we are living through—it is confusion and disorder. On the spiritual plane, pathology is simply being temporarily "disconnected" from God, from the Great Chain of Being and from grace, thus being alienated from Reality both within ourselves and in the world!

In a nutshell, we could say that health is living, growing, maturing. Actualizing our faculties and potentialities, becoming the God-Man we were created to become and thus "doing our duty", "fulfilling our destiny", and "being" what we were meant to be. Whereas illness is its temporary interruption, "getting off our tracks" as it were, becoming blocked, disconnected, and fragmented. Obviously, both health an illness are quite complex and multidimensional phenomena as we are very complex and multidimensional beings!

To preserve our health and avoid illnesses (which, in any case, will also teach us many valuable things), we need to understand the "User's Manual" (see my specific essay on that subject), live by God's laws, and remaining in harmony with our own nature, level of consciousness and evolution, and the environment in which we find ourselves! We need to have faith, live by God's laws, and be positive, happy, and appreciative—remain connected with the ascending spiral and avoid the descending one!

- *Healing*: is the process whereby we restore the lost harmony, peace, justice, connection, and communication both within ourselves and between ourselves and God, Nature, and others human beings. It is part of God's Plan and is already set up to take place both at the *immanent* level (within our bodies and without our consciously seeking to intervene) and at the *transcendent* level (involving our consciousness, choices and actions). It also involves the four essential planes and dimensions of our being, the physical, the emotional, the mental, and the spiritual.

  Interestingly enough, we already have both the *knowledge* (but at the superconscious level) and the *means* (the P.N.E.I axis or psycho-neuro-endocrinological-immune response) to reestablish our health and thus we do not need a complex technology, a sophisticated pharmacopoeia or a lot of money to do so! We need to understand what health, disease, and healing truly are; we also need to get at the underlying causes that brought it about (the "remission of sins"), the removal of the painful symptoms, and the re-establishment of the proper inner harmony and connection. A proper understanding of nutrition, energy and of our destiny!

  Today, in particular, we need to have a proper understanding of the nature and role of energy or *vitality* (as exhaustion or lack of energy is the "mother of all diseases"), of stress and *relaxation* (which is essential for remaining "connected" and preserving the proper "communication lines" with the different aspects and facets of our being and of the world), and of *morality* (namely that the universe is a "mirror" that always sends back to us what we send out in it . . . so that what we do unto others, in the end we do unto ourselves!).

  Specifically, there are certain things that are extremely simple yet profound and indispensable to preserve and restore our health. These are: prayer, fasting, doing what we came in this world to do, helping others through meaningful service and affection, being able to love, to give and receive love-vitamins, and avoiding fear, anxiety and negativity! It is also quite important to have a "family doctor" and a "family Saint", or "Teacher in the invisible worlds", to follow, inspire, and guide us throughout our lives. We should always make our own decision in the end and not delegate these to others, to the so-called experts, as we are responsible for our bodies, our psyches, and our lives, and have come in this world to become *responsible adults*, to make our choices and learn from their consequences! Yet, a "feed-back" and a "sounding board" in a person who is older, wiser, more experienced than we are and who genuinely cares about us could be invaluable and part of the "healing process".

Finally, I would add here that the greatest of all doctors and medicines is *God Himself*, the Spirit Who created us, Who is part of us, and Who loves us so that He will never abandon us and has already given us all that we need to complete our being and fulfill our destiny! Hence, the greatest and most effective remedy is, at the *objective level*, the divine Light, spiritual energies, the *Heilstrom* of Bruno Groening, while at the *subjective level* it is the desire to live, a reason for living, and the energy to be able to do so!

Let me elaborate a little on prayer, fasting, doing what we came to do in this world, helping others and being able to love. First a note a warning and caution. Any healing approach must take into consideration the *level of consciousness and evolution* of the patient . . . and the therapist in order to be truly efficacious and to avoid doing violence to the person. (I have written a book for medical doctors on this subject which I highly recommend for those who want to delve deeper into this fascinating topic, *Medicina Differenziale e Qualitativa*, Guna, 2007).

Obviously, someone who is on a lower of level of consciousness and more physical, needs a more physical approach; someone who is on psychosocial level of consciousness will respond better to psychosomatic or alternative medicine and needs to pay more attention to his/her thoughts and feelings. Finally, a person who seeking or has reached the spiritual level, needs to pay more attention to religious and spiritual means—to prayer, faith, belief systems, and the connection with God. Obviously, this rule also applies to prayer, doing one's duty, helping others, and being able to love . . . even though these have correlations and implications on all levels of consciousness and being.

Prayer implies consciously raising our level of consciousness to the point that we can understand and harmonize with God's Will, that we can establish a conscious "telepathic connection" with the divine Light and the healing energies. Thus it involves the male polarity and "filling oneself up" . . . with

Light, Love, and Life! Fasting is the opposite and complementary process, that deals with the female polarity and which involves "emptying ourselves" so that Something greater and better can fill its place. Thus, there is a physical fasting (not eating or drinking), an emotional fasting (centering ourselves emotionally and avoiding strong positive or negative emotions), a mental fasting (not thinking or emptying our minds of all thoughts and ideas), and a spiritual fasting (listening to the voice of silence, the voice of our higher self). These make us more sensitive and receptive to what exists on these respective levels and helps us "emptying ourselves" so that we can "fill up" with the Light, with God's spiritual energies.

Doing what we came to do in this world, or our "duty", is also a very "simple", powerful and effective remedy in that it helps us harmonize and reconnect with our unconscious (the superconscious in particular) and with the world. By doing this, all the forces within ourselves and in the universe, will help us re-establish the proper connection, circulation and communication with the various parts of our being and of the universe as we are pursuing God's Plan for us and what our soul chose to learn and to achieve in this life. This can greatly vivify and revitalize us as well as help remove blockages.

Helping others and being able *to love* (give and receive love vitamins) is also a very fundamental healing therapy, or healing process, as it draws us out of ourselves, re-establishes lines of communication, vivifies us and makes us feel "alive", makes us forget ourselves and our problems to become fully engrossed in helping others. Love, unquestionably, is the most important ontological attribute of both God and Man and thus goes to the very core of our being and the very essence of Life! In fact, we were created and born to love and when we love, then we want to live, we have a reason for living, and we find the strength and energy to do so! This is the reason why at the very heart of the genuine spiritual life we find *love*, the ability to love God (prayer) others (service) and Life (joy)!

Chapter III

THE ROLE OF RELIGION
AND SPIRITUALITY IN MEDICAL PRACTICE

We have now reached the point in our discussion, analysis and presentation wherein we can get to the very heart or substance of this work: *what could be the role and contribution of religion and spirituality in medical practice?* Are these aspects that must remain separate and distinct from the healing process or are they aspects that we can, fruitfully and demonstrably, integrate in the healing process so as to render them more effective in diminishing human suffering and pain (both on the quantitative and on the qualitative axis)? The answer to this vital question is, once again, paradoxical as it is a function of the level of consciousness and being of the person who provides it. At the personality level, so long as we are dealing with people who are at, or up to, the 3rd level of consciousness and evolution, they should remain *separate* as a distinct specialization. Once we reach the 4th and especially when we access the 5th level, then these must be accounted for and *integrated* as they can make a very major difference.

For let us remember that on the evolutionary path, during the Fall, we are moving from spirit to matter and thus are developing *analysis* and *specialization*. When we reach what I call the 4th level of consciousness and being, which is where the Apocalypse or the great *metanoia*, "conversion and inversion" occur, then we move back from matter to spirit and are learning to make "connections" and integrations of diverse and opposite elements—then we have to "rediscover" and add *synthesis*. Here, there is a profound realization that "all is interconnected and interacting", thus that *everything is important*; that as "above so below" (there are analogies and correspondences on all planes and dimensions of being) and that "only like can know like". Here, we know "scientifically", (i.e. through our own personal experience) that we are multidimensional beings, that there is an evolution of our consciousness, and that on different levels and stages different laws and parameters apply . . . which must be understood and respected.

What this means, practically, is that what might be true and quite important on one level may not be on the next; that as we evolve and raise our consciousness we might have to behave in a different way and thus pay attention to different elements than we did before! What applies to the "baby" and is true for him may not apply and be true for the "child", the "adolescent", the "young adult", etc. Hence, whatever cognitive system we develop in any academic discipline or profession must, necessarily, remain "open" and "dynamic" to *new and emergent elements* and factors. This is particularly true for our bodies, our psyches and souls and thus for our global health! As we move forward in evolution and access higher levels of consciousness and being we need to make the "unconscious conscious" and hence must take into account and integrate new elements and factors, energies and laws with processes that might be antithetical or the opposite of what they were on a lower level.

Today, we know "scientifically" (through mathematics, physics, and biology) that both ourselves and the universe, or what we call "reality", are actually composed of an infinity of energies and frequencies which are multidimensional in nature and which transform themselves, quantitatively and qualitatively, as we rise from plane to plane and access higher levels of consciousness. This can then demonstrate to us that we are truly multidimensional beings living in a multidimensional universe where everything is connected and related to everything else (the Great Chain of Being) and thus that everything is important . . . but some things might be more important than others as they are "causal" or "structuring" to them! This line of connection and causality begins with God, the spirit, to descent to matter . . . and from there to re-ascend to spirit via the psychosocial or human dimension, a growing and unfolding human consciousness.

To ask what might be the "role of religion and spirituality" for our health and wellbeing, hence in an integral medical practice, is to reflect upon what might be the role of ideas, ideologies, thoughts and feelings, of belief systems, and our psychic state of being for our health and well-being, for the proper harmony, circulation, and communication of energies, materials, and information throughout our being. From the standpoint of the spiritual tradition and from the 4th level of consciousness onwards, these become increasingly important and thus play an ever-more significant role, for good as for evil, for healing or for maintaining or even increasing our pathology.

What we need to always keep in mind is that thoughts, feelings, and our overall "state of being" are made up of energies and frequencies that have an impact upon all energies and frequencies, first within our own being and consciousness but then also in the world! As such, they affect all other energies and frequencies to a greater or smaller extent. Thus, they are important and "real" and their impact should grow and intensify with the growth and expansion of our consciousness.

One of the major "problems" or "difficulties" that one encounters here is that of, consciously or unconsciously ", *doing violence* to the other person and projecting one's own views, values, beliefs, and level of consciousness. This is a subtle and complex question but one that needs to be addressed. It involves the ability of our intuition and sympathy to really "tune in to the other person and his/her needs"; the capacity to switch to a "feminine polarity", and the ability to "see" or "respect" the person we are dealing with. These abilities should be part of a program of self-discovery and personal growth.

Thus, to recap: a person is a biological organism, a psychosocial entity, and a spiritual being. All three aspects or levels should be addressed as they have subtle interactions and mutually affect each other. At the conscious and mental level our goal is clearly and unequivocally to bring hope for the mind, motivation for the heart, and energy for the will that will greatly raise that person's energies and frequencies . . . and put them in touch with corresponding ones in their unconscious and in their environment. Religion and spirituality can go a very long ways to achieve this. Religion, however, is still part of the world of duality and can thus be a powerful influence just as much for good as for evil; spirituality, on the other hand, which is part of the world of being and unity and which really begins at the 4th and articulates itself at the 5th level, can either be present or absent and "timing" can be very important as one can seek to introduce it "too soon", when a person is really not yet ready for it as she/he has not yet reached her "spiritual puberty".

To begin with, it is important for the doctor, or health-care practitioner, to understand the "philosophy of life" and the core values and beliefs of those they work with; specifically, I would add, to gage properly where on the "human sky-scraper" that person would fit at present—what is his/her level of consciousness and being? If that person is religious, then it would make sense to approach that person with the perspective and language of his/her religion; if that person is not religious, then it is better not bring in religion and, in particular, not seek to project your religion or to "convert" that person to some of its beliefs and values. The same is true for spirituality! It is important to evaluate whether a person is curious and interested in that approach or not, and if not, then to be very careful not to "shove it down that persons' throat" as it were. It is also very important to be able to render explicit what are that person's greatest *fears, ambiguities and aspirations*. In essence, the key here is to enable the client to take his/her next step in evolution—to make meaningful progress!

Then, slowly and with much delicacy and sensitivity, work together to reframe the mental and emotional state of that person so as to render it much *more positive* and to *integrate opposites, contradictions and negative aspects*; to reframe or "de-dramatize" the situation and seek to point out its positive aspects . . . bearing in mind the very simple but profound Spanish proverb that comes straight from the spiritual tradition, "No y mal che por bien no venga" (there is no evil that does not come for some good). The goal here being to lead that person, by degrees, to reacquire faith in himself/herself, in Life and in a Greater Power; to show, both in theory and by examples, that there are no "hopeless situations" and that there is always, in all situations, *some progress that can be made*, something that can make that person a better person than he/she was before!

It is profound wisdom and also common sense and repeated experience that shows how, many times, it is not possible for as person to change his outer, material, objective situation, but that it is always possible for that person to change his perception, definition, and reaction to a given objective situation. This is an area where modern medicine, both allopathic and alternative, has much to learn and where religion and spirituality have truly major contributions to make. If people can understand what is going on (diagnosis or global evaluation), if they have some feelings as to where it is leading to (prognosis), it can make it much easier to be patient, to accept a given situation, and to cooperate with the treatment or cure; and this is what conventional healthcare generally provides for its patients.

However, maybe even more important than the a diagnosis and prognosis is the ability to *make sense*, to perceive meaning, purpose and value, and *to understand* what one is presently going through; to know that things do not happen by chance, hazard, good or bad luck, that there is a cause and effect relationship in whatever one is experiencing; and that, somehow, one will benefit from the experience that one is living through, that it will enrich us, help us learn, grow, and mature—that it is *not in vain*! And this is the area where religion and spirituality can, indeed, make very fundamental and distinctive contributions! More and more people want to understand, to make sense, and to find meaning and value in what they are living through and this "meaning" and "value" are not something that a technical approach, however efficient, can provide.

For this will immediately change a person's "state of mind", the way they are thinking and feeling about themselves and what they are experiencing. And this, in turn, will have an immediate impact upon their *Vis Medicatrix Naturae* or P.N.E.I. axis as it is called today. This brings to mind what F. Nietzsche once stated, which was picked up by Viktor Frankel and which became the foundation of his school of psychotherapy, Logotherapy, namely: "whenever people have a "why" they can then bear any "how""; in other words, so long as they can perceive meaning purpose and value in their experience, they can live through it and will not crack up psychologically. But, should that "meaning, purpose, and value" disappear, then even minor problems, pains and sufferings will make them "fall apart", dissociate their personality, simply "give up", "rebel", become aggressive towards others or towards themselves, or seek addictive and negative "escapes from reality".

This is the reason why it is so important for people to have a "religion", a "philosophy of life", or a set of assumptions, that will enable them to make sense out of their experiences and lead them to conclude that life is, indeed, WORTHWILE, no matter how hard, painful, unjust, or crazy it might become.

At least for some, this might be even more important than finding a technical solution to their problems and eliminating their painful and dysfunctional symptoms! And this is what the new paradigm in medicine, the integral medicine and the doctor of the future, will have to provide or help his clients to discover and put together! To put this in other words, people need a *trans-empirical frame of reference* that takes into account not only what happens in this life, but in their entire evolution; they need to be able to focus on what is eternal and not just temporal, of this world! And this is what religion and spirituality can do at their best and is their distinct characteristic and contribution!

Since a human being is a sentient being it is essential for him to find and articulate an anthropology, a cosmology, and a theology that will help him link and explain his present condition at the physical, human, and spiritual levels. This is what religions have always provided, in a symbolic and analogical way, and what authentic spirituality can provide at an experiential level: to come up with meaningful answers to the questions "who am I"? "What is the universe in which I live?", "What is Life all about?" and "Why do we have to go through and experience death and birth, health and illness, and experience good and evil?" But to do so, they must take into account the *level of consciousness and evolution* of the person they are dealing with so as not do violence to their personality (i.e. expect a baby to act like a child, a child like an adolescent, or an adolescent like an adult). And this is the reason why the medicine of the future will have to be a "differential and qualitative one" that takes into account not only the horizontal, quantitative dimension but also the vertical, qualitative one.

Here, we also find two basic ways of intervening: by what *one does and say* and by what *one is and radiates*! Many times, it is more important to be relaxed, hopeful, joyful, and vibrantly alive than saying profound things or prescribing a whole array of tests and therapies! For this speaks directly to a person's unconscious and does not require a special attention, interest or cognitive skills! Thus it can be applied to very young, very old and very sick persons. There is also an innate tendency in human beings to imitate and seek to become like the persons they admires and looks up to. This is also an unconscious or subconscious trait but a powerful and deeply ingrained one. Especially in children and young persons this is very evident, as it is when a person has a teacher or a doctor they depend upon and respect! The healthcare specialist will send many messages and communicate on different levels with the persons they are working with, all of which are important and can make a difference.

In conclusion, the doctor will have to assume several role relationships for his clients (healer, teacher, priest, advocate, friend, etc.) and be able to switch from the female (receptive) to the male (directive) polarity. First, he needs to really "look at" and "understand" his patient, have genuine sympathy and empathy with him together with the belief that he can help in a significant way and have the desire to do so. In simple words, he has to learn *to love* and be able *to communicate* with the patient. As we are moving forward in our evolution and as we raise our level of consciousness and being even further, it is important that both patient and doctor feel that it is their "destiny" to work together, that there is a link and a bond between them that is mutual! Thus the present universalistic approach will have to be moderated and deepened with a more particularistic one.

As I pointed out in other writings and lectures, there is a spectrum amongst healthcare professionals that is quite specific and important and it is not by "chance" or "hazard" that a person will end up with one or the other of the three types . . . and, obviously, this will make an enormous difference! In the middle of that scale and covering the vast majority of persons (80%-90%) we have *professionals* who are giving a service for pay. Like everyone else in this world, they have to make a living, they have to study, and they have to provide a valuable service and be paid for it. These can be better or worse and specialize in one or another field, but they give a service for which they are paid. And again, some may be more or less concerned with the financial aspect of this arrangement and work with more or less wealthy clients. On the whole today, given the length of the studies involved to get a license and given the aptitudes and talents that are required, healthcare professionals, medical doctors in particular, will aspire to an upper middle class or middle class way of life . . . that their patients have to pay for.

At the bottom, we have the "sharks", i.e. ambitious and greedy persons who realize that a sick or suffering person will pay whatever they can afford to be healed and be rid of their pains. Again, these maybe more or less technically competent and more or less skillful in their specialty, but their overriding and ultimate goal remain *financial and professional success*. And this they generally obtain . . . with some of them who can actually make fortunes which, today, can amount to millions! While they maybe technically quite competent and even brilliant, the quality of the service they render is very different from that of the other two types . . . and generally patients will eventually sense and become aware of this and seek better help elsewhere!

At the top of the scale with have what I call the "missionaries", i.e. those who really feel they have come in this world to heal the sick and diminish human suffering and who will do this even if it costs them many efforts, sacrifices and deprivations, and if they are poorly or not remunerated! I do not have specific statistics on the "sharks" and the "missionaries", but they are definitely in a small minority. At the top of this type, we find the great Saints, Sages, and genuine Healers who can practice "spiritual medicine at its best" and obtain sensational or what is generally called "miraculous" healings with practically "nothing" (no professional training, degrees, licenses, or clinical experience)! Good examples of these might be Padre Pio, Jean Vianney, and Brother André who were in religious orders and eventually canonized. Non-religious examples would be Maître Philippe de Lyons, Rita Cutolo, and Bruno Groening who, while not particularly religious, were profoundly spiritually oriented.

Every race, every religion, every part of the world at all times have had a few such individuals who have appeared, done their work, and then left . . . but left having healed a large number of people of practically all kinds of diseases, and this either gratuitously or for very little money. I was fortunate in my life to meet and experience a few such people and thus got a "living model" of the fact that they do exist and that they can truly perform outstanding cures (provided that this is in the destiny of the recipient) and outstanding healings in most cases. Not too long ago, I have wondered how many people, on a percentage basis in a given country, get to meet with such a person—which is a very small percentage and certainly less than 1%? Then, I wondered why these few were so "lucky" to make such an encounter? I finally came to the double conclusion that this also does not happen by "hazard" but is part of the "destiny" of the person to whom it happens to have that privilege; and that one can actually "earn" or "prepare" for that privilege . . . by working upon oneself, raising one's level of consciousness, and actively seeking to help others!

Thus as the spiritual tradition has always taught, it is never by "chance" that a student ends up with a given professor, a doctor or a healer with a given patient, and a husband with a given wife and vice versa! Human beings are truly multidimensional beings who act like *magnets* (but yet mainly unconsciously) to attract the kinds of people and experiences . . . they need at that level of consciousness and being for their own growth and self-actualization. This is the "esoteric" or hidden reason why one should *never blame others* but always *work upon one's self* to raise one's level of consciousness and being and to grow and mature, because it is only in this way that one can meet "better" or more evolved persons!

I had the privilege of experiencing and "testing out" at least three times in my life in a very major way what it could mean to "meet the right person at the right time" to get out of an impasse and to take one's next step in evolution. These encounters, which were part of my destiny and a great gift of Heaven also led to me understand and experience what religion and spirituality could do for a person in very difficult circumstances. Finally, they led me to understand "experientially" the difference and complementarity between priests and prophets, between the clergy who has the "letter" of the tradition and the initiate who has the "spirit" of that tradition; these also led me to live and experience personally the fact that no situation is ever "completely helpless", that one is never given "a cross heavier than what one can bear", and that all human experiences can be transformed into spiritual opportunities for growth and self-actualization; or, in one sentence, that *life is always worthwhile!* And this, most of the time, not so much by changing one's external circumstances as by "reframing them", by looking at them from a *different angle*, by changing one's own way of perceiving, defining, and reacting to them!

When I was yet very young and just beginning to become aware of myself and of the world in which I found myself, I looked upon life on earth as the *worst possible hell*—as a madhouse and a battlefield—where the craziest things take place and where, most of the time, one must face and deal with the three faces evil: lies, violence, and ugliness or disharmony . . . and this when one has just gone "amnesiac", having lost one's true identity and the awareness of the real purpose for being born in this world! Thus, my first real "prayer" or "cry of my heart" was "O God, take me back home, make me die as soon as possible". But, obviously, this was not possible and I had to stay here and go on with my life . . . and to do that in a truly "real and meaningful fashion" I had to *find people to help me* (even though I did not have the faintest idea as to "who" they were or how to "find them" in this world) and I had to find a rational understanding, meaning, purpose and value in what I was confronted with and had to live through.

In retrospect, but certainly not at the time I was going through some of the more difficult and painful experiences of my life, I discovered that there is a "providence", which is exceedingly wise, loving, and powerful, which is at work in our lives and that, indeed, what seems "impossible for men" is quite possible for God! These people did "find me" and we did meet, in various places and countries and on various levels. I was provided with both the *knowledge* and the *tools* or means to do what I had come here to do. These things, however, were not "given to me on a silver platter" or "done for me", I had to do them! What I was given was the knowledge and understanding, the motivation and desire, and finally the energy and the strength to do "my duty" and fulfill my purpose.

Essentially, the Saints and Sages, the most important and significant persons I met all had a "gift for me" but a gift that I had to "work on" and utilize if I wanted to benefit from what it could contribute to me. In various ways and through different paths, as I have mentioned in the former parts of this work and in other works, I was led to religion and spirituality as the true "fountain head" of the *knowledge, love and life* I sought. Science and education, to which I dedicated my life, were also very important, but they turned out to be more "means" than "ends", a method and a philosophy, I could use to solve the truly fundamental questions of life.

After having been very disappointed and "turned off by my own religion" (because it was not what I expected it to be and because it did not do for me what I thought I needed and wanted), I came back to religion and integrated spirituality in it as well as in other academic and professional fields such as education, sociology, psychology, psychotherapy and medicine. Thus, I personally lived the fact that "a little knowledge takes one away from God while a lot of knowledge brings one back to God". This led me, moreover, to discover, as I mentioned several times, that religion does have the "answers" and the "tools" through which one can answer the fundamental questions of life; not the "exoteric" but "esoteric" aspect of religion; not institutionalized religion but the religion of the Saints and Sages that can link the "letter" with the "spirit" and make that religion truly alive.

The first thing that I "discovered" and became aware of is that there are, indeed, men and women in this world who have a far greater knowledge and powers than what most people think and could even imagine. Some of these things you have to see and experience for yourself in order to believe and accept them for they do seem to contradict and negate what we take for granted and our so-called "scientific vision" of the world! Then, I was given the "explanatory key" of symbolic and analogical language or the ability to look at archetypes and to begin interpreting them on different levels of consciousness. At a rudimentary level, I was also given the insight of the human sky-scraper and the vertical axis of consciousness.

More important, around the time when I was 20 years old, I received the insight of the "microcosm-macrocosm analogy" (i.e. that whatever exists or happens in the world has to exist and take place within ourselves so that external worldly personages and events must now be interpreted in internal, psychological entities and processes). And this led me to mystical or "esoteric Christianity" which provided the link with the other traditions and the inner keys for understanding and living that tradition.

Around that period of time, I also began to experience physical and psychological symptoms that official medicine could not understand and was certainly not able to resolve for me. This led me to travel to Paris and to discover "alternative and spiritual medicine", thus opening another "door" for me. A few years later, I had my motorcycle accident which was, unquestionably, one of the most important and formative incidents of my life. For a fairly long period of time (about 30 months) my life was really thrown "up-side-down"; I was told by the best medical authorities that I could not possibly heal that that I would remain crippled for the rest of my life. And this made it absolutely and physically impossible for me to fulfill my purpose and destiny . . . which I had discovered at the age of 15 and which had led me to the United States . . .

For a while "reality became a nightmare for me and my dreams became reality". At that time, even though I had met some authentic Sages and Saints, I still believed in conventional medicine and thought that science was a slow but incontrovertible path to "truth" and "reality", thus I was devastated and, once again, hoped I would die as soon as possible . . . and even thought of doing away with my body which had become a "prison" and which prevented me from being what I was and doing what I had come in this world to do! One thing, however, did remain: I remembered that Einstein had stated repeatedly (which I learned in my physics courses at Columbia university) that "all human problems have a solution, but that solution many times could only be found on a *higher level* than the problem and not on the same level". My "problem", as I then defined it, was to discover and understand *why* that bloody accident had occurred to me as I also believed that "nothing happens by "hazard" or "random chance".

It is here that religion and spirituality really came into my life at a very personal and essential level. Of all the means I could have used to raise my consciousness to that "higher level" (and there were many of different types and approaches) I chose *prayer*. I chose prayer because I had already seen some of its powers and potentialities and was able to rationally grasp some of its processes and possibilities. Thus, I turned to *religion* (the Eastern Orthodox Christian tradition, the most mystical of the three branches of Christianity) as the "essential means" and to *spirituality* (the activation of the intuition, the awakening of spiritual consciousness, and access to the reign of grace) as the "fundamental end". For about six months, I used various techniques and approaches I had gathered prior to my accident from various people, traditions, and systems, but without any tangible results . . . Then the concrete and practical results began to take place in the simplest and most natural way.

First, I began to finally *accept* (with my heart as well as my head) the fact that I would remain crippled for the rest of my life and thus that I could not "fulfill my destiny", but that I could still have a very meaningful life, learn many important things, and make real progress. Then, I became slowly aware that that accident had been an intrinsic and very important *part of my destiny* which, however and for obvious reasons, was not revealed to me at the age of 15 when I became aware of my overall destiny or what I had come to achieve in this world. Lastly, I also became aware that, in fact, what was deemed "impossible" by the medical-scientific world was in fact "possible"; namely that I could heal and have a "normal life" after all which would enable me to return to the United States and to continue with my life where I had "left off"!

Somehow (and I feel this was also part of the Plan and of my destiny), it took a "long time" for me to realize that I could heal just as it took a "long time" (about 18 months for the first most difficult phase and 2-3 years to fully complete the process) for me to fully heal. During those crucial 3-5 years when the major "turn-about occurred", religion and spirituality played an absolutely vital role for me. Without them I honestly do not know what would have happened, what I would have done or what turn my life would have taken. Religion and spirituality helped me in three essential ways that I believe could be *generalized and applied to other persons* as well: first they gave me a *perspective* and a *belief system* that enabled me to make sense out of what I was going through at the time. Secondly, they gave me the *support system* (people and love) to help me and encourage me when I would "go down". Thirdly they gave me *access to the energy and strength to keep going*.

To state it synthetically, they enable me to access higher laws, energies and frequencies than those that are known and used by present day science and they provided me with a trans-empirical frame of reference that enabled me to focus not only on the temporal things of this world in one life-time but also on eternal things that involve our entire evolution and being.

Chapter IV

CORE CONTRIBUTIONS OF RELIGION AND SPIRITUALITY TO THE MEDICAL PROFESSION AND HEALTHCARE IN GENERAL

As we have seen, religion and spirituality, which are functions of our level of consciousness and being and which can therefore manifest in very different ways (with genuine spirituality appearing only on the 4th level of consciousness), can make very significant contributions to human beings both on the generic level of well-being and on the specific level of healthcare. If we try to systematize these, here is what we find (which I suggest you reflect upon, personalize, and apply in your own lives and professions):

Religion offers a *belief system* which is trans-empirical focused on a larger picture of life that enables us to look at things and events *sub species temporalis* and especially *sub* species *aeternitatis* (i.e. including both the temporal and the eternal aspects). As such, this belief system can help us "reframe" difficult situations, develop patience and acceptance, with the realization that we are not "victims" of a blind, indifferent or hostile, fate and that we can benefit from all that happens to us and that we live through *without exceptions*. It also offers a *ritual system* whereby we can tap and experience some of the higher energies, laws and frequencies, access the "realm of grace", and climb on the inner sky-scraper.

It offers us an *ethical system* with specific guidelines as to what is "good" or "bad" for us and for our relationships with things and beings outside of ourselves; basically, it shows us that the universe is really a "mirror" that sends back to us what we send out to it and that what we do unto others, ultimately we do unto ourselves . . . as we are all interconnected and interrelated. It provides us with a *social organization* system whereby we learn how we can enter into meaningful and lawful relationships with others. Lastly, it is also supposed to provide us

234

with *personal experience system* whereby we can not only "read about, hear, and believe in certain things" but also *experience them*. And, in my opinion, this is the weak point of the Western institutionalized religions which are barely able to do this at the present time and which is the reason why they pushes aspiring souls to other religions or schools.

In view of the foregoing, it is clear that religion is a part of our human culture, the way in which we organize, develop and manifest our human consciousness. As such, it helps is to create cosmos out of chaos, both in the microcosm, at the psychological level, and in the macrocosm, at the sociocultural world; how to provide order, structure, and motivation for us to continue our growth and evolution process. It is still part of the world of duality and of phenomena, of our personality, but it can lead us by degree to the world of unity and of noumena, of our soul, by creating an interdimensional "channel" or communication line. This "bridge" can help us to go on when through our own efforts we could not as we gave and did all that we could! Religion therefore, can help us bridge and united human effort and divine grace and lead us from the world to nature to access the world of grace, thereby accelerating our evolution and leading us, by degree and in an organic fashion, to the 4th and 5th level of consciousness where spirituality—which is its end—can be born!

Spirituality is the process and the great goal which will lead us to finally discover experientially who we are, where we come from, where we are going, what we came in this world to achieve and what is our "duty" and "destiny" in this world—it will lead us to discover and experience our Self and God, the Ultimate Reality both, internally and externally! It will lead us to the "Kingdom of God" (genuine spiritual consciousness) and to the "Heavenly Jerusalem" (our superconscious wherein our spiritual Self, or divine spark, dwells). Hence, it will help us, at long last, answer the truly fundamental questions of life and be able to know, be, and express ourselves and to truly LIVE, consciously and fully, focusing upon and realizing what is truly essential and what we really came to do in this world. From the 5th level of consciousness and being it will lead us to the 6th and 7th at which point incarnation in this physical world will no longer be necessary as we will have accomplished all that life on earth can offer! But we may choose to return, once again, freely and without necessity, to help humankind on its long journey back home!

More specifically, spirituality will help us create the order and structure, both at the cognitive and at the existential level, to bring together all the various fragmented parts of our consciousness, knowledge, activities and being. As such it will bring religion, healthcare, education, as well as all the other academic disciplines, vocations and professions, to the *5th level of consciousness, being and evolution* wherein a genuine unity, synthesis, and interrelationship can meaningfully take place. In summary and in simple words, it will lead us to realize that Life and all that it entails, with its myriad of experiences and adventures, is truly WORTHWHILE and that it does lead somewhere, which is far more magnificent and wondrous than anything we could ever have thought or imagined on lower levels of consciousness. And thus that all our efforts, all our mistakes and sufferings, all our sacrifices and aspirations were not in vain. This truly is something which must be personally experienced to be understood as there are no words or points of reference that can take its place and do justice to what it represents.

Coming now to the level of medicine, healthcare and wellbeing, religion and spirituality have very major and distinctive contributions to make which can immeasurably contribute to alleviate human suffering and pain, restore and maintain health and joy, and help us fulfill the purpose for which we were born in this troubled and confusing world. It is most important, however, to put them into proper perspective and to be clear as to what they can and what they cannot do. Both will affect, first, foremost and primarily, the second aspect of our being, the human or psychosocial one, our *human consciousness*, or way of perceiving, defining, and reacting to "reality". But they will also have a "feed-back-loop" and affect, but indirectly, our physical or biological being and our spiritual being. To put it in a nutshell, they will enable us to *transform and raise our consciousness* to the point wherein we can again make sense and cope with whatever life is throwing at us.

They will affect our *vitality level* by affecting our energy-bodies and their psychospiritual centers which, in turn, will have a profound impact upon our physical body and our soul. This will reactivate and harmonize our bio-psycho-spiritual harmony, our inner and outer interaction and communication, so that our P.N.E.I axis (the immune, hormonal, nervous, and circulatory systems) can do their work of self-repair and the proper maintenance of our bodies. They will also enable our consciousness and being, again through our energy-bodies and their psychospiritual centers, to remain "connected" and thus able to make exchanges with our spiritual Self and our superconscious . . . which will provide the energy, guidance, and motivation so that we can fulfill our purpose in this world!

The fundamental goals and objectives of the 5th level of medicine, spiritual medicine, are very simple and clear, but it is important to keep them in mind and not claim that they can do other than what they are meant and structured to accomplish. These are to bring *peace of mind, serenity, acceptance, appreciation and gratitude*—a new and different state of being for both the patient and the doctor. It is not the aim of spiritual medicine to cure the patient and thus full healing cannot be promised or presented as the end. God, the cooperation, and motivation of the patient, together with his/her present situation and destiny, will bring this about . . . or will not bring it about!

But, if the connection, relationship, and work that are undertaken by both is done correctly, there can and there will be a "reframing" of the client's situation and a different way of perceiving, defining, and reacting to his situation. Thus healing will occur at the spiritual and psychological level. According to a number of complex and highly personalized variables these may well bring about a "cure" or the extinction of the painful and dysfunctional symptoms with their underlying pathology . . . or it may not! For the normal and healthy state of a person is to be well, conscious, vital and joyful and not afflicted by fatigue, inflammation, infection, fever or pain!

Most important here is to keep in mind that genuine healing always moves from the inside out, from above below, and retraces the same course that did the illness. Thus, some time may be necessary for full healing and being cured—which could vary from a few seconds to a few years! By changing our level of consciousness, our perception and attitude towards our illness, we will, sooner and later and in one fashion or another, also affect that illness at the physical level. This because the body reflects the psyche as the psyche reflects the soul: all are interconnected as they are also interconnected with their "world" or environment.

Another important factor here is the so called "Herxheimer effect" or therapeutic worsening as we work with and invoke spiritual energies and higher frequencies. This is probably the best and surest sign that "something is happening" and that the client is receiving the healing light and higher frequencies. Bruno Groening and his Circle of Friends call this *Regelung (en)* which in German means "regulation" or *restoring order*. Both Bruno Groening and the spiritual tradition have argued that pathology is evil (but that evil always works, in the end, to bring about good . . . but in an unconscious and unwanted way!) and that an important aspect or expression of both pathology and evil is *disorder*. Hence healing really implies and brings about the restoration of *order* (both within the individual and in his environment).

This "healing crisis" involves a process of "detoxification", inner cleaning and re-harmonization, which entails getting rid of negative elements and re-establishing a new harmony and line of communication. It is most important that persons who are seeking help from 4th and 5th level medicine (which includes *causes* and not only the removal of *symptoms*) be prepared for that and do not interpret it as a "regression" or "worsening of the illness". It is the surest sign that the higher energies and frequencies are at work, that that the healing process is underway, but that patience and perseverance are also needed.

Schematizing and summarizing this process, we can look for and expect the following manifestations:

1. The symptoms and pains move from the inside of the body to the outside (a Herpes Zoster inflammation could move from the lungs or the trigeminal nerves to the skin and flare up as "shingles").

2. The symptoms move from the upper part of the body to the lower (head or chest pains caused by food or drug intoxication could now "move out" by causing pain and swelling in the legs or feet).

3. The symptoms of a chronic illness will begin disappearing in the *inverse order of their appearance*; thus the last ones will be the first to leave and the first ones may, once again, appear and be the last to be extinguished. This could also be due to the fact that symptoms that were denied or repressed could reappear again when a person undertakes a healing process that is natural and integral. Thus their reappearance is really the best sign or "signal" of the self-healing of the body.

4. Generally, the "therapeutic worsening" may be preceded by a generalized and profound sensation of well-being, a feeling that authentic healing is finally taking place.

5. At times, this sense of "profound and inner well-being" may occur even during the "therapeutic worsening process", indicating that at the higher levels and in the depths of our being *changes are taking place* which are very positive and leading in the right direction.

The most common and basic symptoms of this "therapeutic worsening process" or "healing crisis" can be summarized as follows:

o   A sensation of general fatigue weakness and coldness.
o   Diverse pains and discomfort including muscular pains.
o   Fever, shaking, bleeding and cough.
o   Frequent urination or sweating.
o   Unusual bodily odors and skin irruptions.
o   Diarrhea or constipation.
o   A temporary disappearance of sexual desire.
o   Digestive or stomach and colon pains.
o   Emotional symptoms such as irritability, reactivity, anxiety, fears, and sadness.
o   Sleep disturbances such as nightmares, insomnia, or prolonged periods of sleep and sleepiness.

Other symptoms may other manifest themselves as these are highly personalized reactions to a wide variety of problems and disharmonies.

A final but most important point here is the following: remember that you cannot give that which you do not are or are not! Thus at the spiritual level, it is important for the doctor or healthcare practitioner to prepare himself/herself, to raise his/her level of consciousness, to *pray regularly* for and with the patient, and to be upbeat and joyful when meeting with the patient. As the aim here is to convey hope, motivation, and life; to radiate and exemplify peace of mind, serenity, acceptance, appreciation, and gratitude; it is essential that the therapist can integrate, live and radiate these qualities for the patient who will enter in resonance with the therapist.

In the end what will happen is that the healthcare practitioner will become not only a "technician" but also a "healer"; namely that he/she will become the *greatest healing instrument and medicine* for the patient by what he/she is and what he/she radiates—by the Light and Love he/she can manifest! This Light and Love which are the tangible manifestation of the Ultimate Reality will restore order, harmony, and communication or what we call health, wellbeing, and joy!

Chapter V

HOW TO INTEGRATE RELIGION AND SPIRITUALITY IN ONE'S LIFE AND PROFESSION?

The answer here is quite simple and self-evident: *you must live and be* what you are trying to do and teach others! But we must also realize that everyone is not on the same level of consciousness and being that you are; that there exist several different levels of consciousness and beings each of which has its own distinctive modalities and characteristics which must be understood and respected. One has every right (and, in fact, also the duty) to be what one is and to function of the level of consciousness one is functioning on.

One of the essential goals of the spiritual path is none other than "building character and integrity" which means "being true to one's self"! But these may be different, even opposed for different people. Hence, it is most important not to do violence to oneself or to one's clients, to be sensitive to their own needs, aspiration, and levels, and to be motivated to help them "take the next step" in their growth and evolution. For the spiritual tradition, it is this that being able to truly "love" one's patient will accomplish . . . as love activates sympathy and empathy and enhances intuition, inspiration and the life forces in both parties!

An interesting point here is that when we reach the 4th and 5th level of consciousness and evolution, we come to the paradoxical conclusion that we need to have a "religion", a basic cognitive structure and practical rule for our lives; but that we can also understand and deal with people who do not have or feel the need for a religion, or that have a different "religion" or "philosophy of life" than our own. At that point, we begin to really understand the image of the human sky-scraper, to acquire a sense of self-worth and inner security that comes from our own conscience and, therefore, we can be much more tolerant and understanding of others who are on a different level than our own.

Perhaps even more important, we have a made a subtle but essential switch from knowledge and power to love and compassion. What is really essential, our "salvation" as it were, will not come from having gathered a great deal of knowledge or being able to wield different and awesome powers, but from being able *to love*, to establish right relationships, to truly be capable of understanding, feeling, with and wanting to help others. Thus, we will begin to realize that the first and most important thing we can do for others (that a therapist can do for his patients) is to *work on himself and raise his level of consciousness* . . . to access those levels where the true answers can, indeed, come from.

The "means" is religion but the "end" is spirituality; the picture can be very beautiful and useful but it is not the person or object it represents and, sooner or later, must lead us to the latter. If the transformation and expansion of consciousness is the essential process and solution to the human dilemma, direct personal experience is the foundation and substance of that process. Thus anyone who wants to help others, in whatever capacity and for whatever reason, must begin working upon one's self. This entails two fundamental aspects: the *cognitive* (knowledge, understanding, awareness) and the practical-existential (the actual living or experience). Religion has always been the "means" to provide both because *homo sapiens* is truly *homo religiosus*; that is a being who seeks to bring fragments and disconnected parts together in a coherent "whole"; a being who seeks meaning and purpose, a being who seeks what is real and thus worthwhile and this not only at a conscious but also at a superconscious and unconscious level, in the heights and depths of his being.

This means that "religion", a philosophy and art of living, that are in sync with one's being and level of consciousness, is fundamental; that it is more than worth all the time, energy and travail dedicated to finding it and to living it! It is important, however, to always keep one's mind, heart and will focused on the ultimate end and grand goal: *full and conscious union with God*, the perfection of our being, the actualization of our faculties and potentialities and the realization of our destiny. There are different roads and paths that lead there and, in ultimate analysis, all roads lead there for there is nothing that is absolutely evil or wasted, but the paths can be quite different with different implications. As one grows and matures, one will become more tolerant and understanding of others and more demanding and strict with one's self . . .

A most important help in the process of achieving our goal and of attaining real success is to be able to encounter and interact with persons who are on a higher level of consciousness and being than one's own, to know and interact with Saints and Sages. Then, in turn, on a lower level and in a more modest way, the doctor or therapist will be able to provide the same for his patients—a living "model" and "example", a mobile "fountain of love vitamins", and a dynamic source of health, life and joy! The message that that person will then convey to others and to her patients in particular, is: look what you can become, look at the opportunities and treasures of life, it is really worth living to the fullest . . . and here is the knowledge, the companionship, and the means to do so!

In a nutshell this is my vision of the "doctor of the future" and of the "medicine of the future". It will be a lot less dangerous, a lot more simple and natural, a lot less expensive, and far more effective than anything we have come up with so far. More important, it will co-involve at a very vital level the *cooperation of the patient*, his motivation, and desire to get well and stay well, for this is the only way that he will be able to fully make use of the great opportunity for self-discovery, self-improvement, and self-realization which is life on earth! It will also help the patient become responsible, autonomous, and self-reliant so that a new type of relationship, a more "symmetrical" or equal type of relationship can be established between therapist and client, the type of relationship which is best described by the word "amitié" (friendship) and which in French clearly and unequivocally points to the soul (âme) and a relationship between souls!

Conclusion

In the third part of this work, I have sought to focus our attention upon the role of religion and spirituality for the healthcare, wellness, and holistic religion of the future and to get us to reflect and meditate upon some of the basic implications and applications it might have for all of us. After discussing and examining what religion and spirituality are and how they relate to our present level of consciousness and being, I have suggested that, today, they will really "come unto their own", experience a true and major Renaissance, and become much more important and less ambiguous, conflictual and paradoxical than they have been in the last three centuries and still are today.

My basic thesis, in fact, is that they are truly essential and have no valid "functional substitutes" if we are to discover our true identity and destiny and be able to realize both. To do so, however, we need to grow and mature, we need to raise our level of consciousness and evolution to the 4th and then the 5th level where religion will have to bring together and unite the "letter" with the "spirit", its exoteric with its esoteric aspects, and the "religion of the masses" with that of the Saints and Sages. For religion, the "means", this is particularly important as its beliefs, symbols, rites, and teachings can articulate and manifest themselves on all seven level of consciousness and being, and can be used just as much for good as they can for evil—for facilitating and accelerating our evolution . . . or for slowing it down and hampering it!

For spirituality, the "end", really emerges and comes into being, in a full, conscious, and authentic way, only at the 4th and 5th level and is thus "missing" or "latent" until that time. Thus, it demands a certain level of evolution, maturity and consciousness before it can really become a "real" and "living" force in our lives and consciousness. Now, unless I am mistaken, the time for this to occur is precisely today, the end of the 20th and the beginning of the 21st century!

When we move from privileging knowledge and will to giving priority to love and relationships, when we pass from the era of having to the era of being, then we will "rediscover" and reintegrate synthesis with analysis and seek to aim at what is essential, what is meaningful, what is real—and this always implies what is connected, interacting, and united not what is separated, alienated, and fragmented! Then, we shall become aware that medicine and healthcare are not only specialties but also part of the whole, of our entire lives and of all important cognitive pursuits.

Applying our two central explanatory keys, the parable of the Prodigal Son and the theory of the human sky-scraper, our long pilgrimage in the physical world and our different levels of consciousness to the role of religion and spirituality in healthcare, we can get some very interesting insights and make very useful associations. Healthcare and the art of living began by being the *part of an interconnected and interacting whole* where everything was related to everything else and where wisdom consisted in being able to focus upon what was really essential and thus effective and useful. In primitive and traditional societies, which retained a close connection with the vertical dimension and the spiritual realm, the doctor or therapist was also the priest, the educator, the advocate and the friend—he was someone that knew, understood, cared for, respected you and could help with the difficult *art of living*. In turn, he was highly respected and esteemed and would be helped in return by his community and constituents.

With the Fall and the downward thrust of involution, we moved from unity to diversity and multiplicity, we made analysis and specialization primary and thus lost the understanding and recognition of the importance of interrelationships—we learned more and more about less and less! We developed specialized technicians who developed very sophisticated theories and complex technologies which, however, became less and less effective in preserving or restoring integral health. With Redemption, the great "inversion" or "turn-around" and the upward thrust of evolution, we are now moving from matter back to spirit and thus from multiplicity, separation, and fragmentation to unity, connectedness, and wholeness (from the infinite number of illnesses to the one integral health). Thus, we are re-discovering the importance of synthesis, of love and relationships and of multidimensionality . . . which implies profound modesty and humility in front of reality.

Hence, in all fields, we are seeking not only or exclusively *scientific knowledge* but also and on an increasing scale, *wisdom*. Wisdom consists in blending human effort with divine grace, the male with the female principle, objectivity with subjectivity, and knowledge and thought with love and feeling; wisdom is also traveling on the opposite path of scientific knowledge namely aiming at becoming simpler, more natural, less expensive, and more effective because truly rooted in "reality"! Here religion, as the means, and spirituality, which is the end, will play a truly fundamental role with distinctive contributions that have no substitute.

Here, the healthcare specialist or doctor will also have to become the healer: priest, teacher, and friend, he will become the Sage and the Saint who will be most effective in helping people access their own resources and potentialities, to reconnect with God, and thus to be able to achieve their destiny in this world and live more *abundant* and *conscious lives* . . . which means to live in a more responsible, autonomous, productive healthy, moral, creative, and joyful way where love will prevail and predominate!

Conclusion

This work was originally conceived to be published in three volumes, each dealing with a specific topic that remained intimately connected with the other two. After further reflection and discussion with a few friends, praying and meditating about this, I decided to publish it in one volume but with three distinct and particular parts which complement and complete each other. Religion has always been a very major cognitive and moral anchor, a social institution which played a key role for all human beings to create cosmos out of chaos both at the inner, psychological level, and at the outer, environmental level. It has provided a set of symbols, myths and rites through which human beings could begin to make sense (from their growing consciousness and awareness) that they had to be able to structure, *interpret and explain the human condition*, but the meaning, implications and applications of which could and have greatly changed in different times and places. Thus human beings have been rightly defined as a *homo religiosus*, a religious being!

Endowed with physical, psychological and spiritual needs and aspirations, human beings had the difficult task of learning how to survive in the physical world, then how to live well, and finally and most importantly, to understand why they were born in this world and what they were meant to accomplish here—what was their "duty" and destiny" that would enable them to the most conscious, productive and meaningful life. On the various levels of consciousness, being and evolution, with perhaps the exception of the 3rd level which corresponds to what I call the "person of talent" or the "adolescent" (who rebels against tradition and custom and who wants to become "independent", autonomous, and make his own personal experiences from which to draw his basic conclusions), religion has always played a very central role in human affairs.

However, as I tried to point out and demonstrate, religion can only be a "means", a scaffolding, a basic perspective and set of tools that will lead us to the true "end" which is spirituality, which must be grounded in direct personal experience, and which emerges at the 4th level to fully articulate itself only at the 5th level of consciousness and being. Today we know from history and experience in various fields and sectors of life that the "means" can be transformed into the "end", which then disappears, and that there is always a dialectic tension between the "means" (religion and the clergy) and the "end" (spirituality and mystics, Saints and Sages).

Thus I felt that the time had come, in the development of my own thinking and life, as well as at the external, cultural and historical period we are now living in, to focus upon both religion and spirituality to see how these would "appear": be looked at, defined, and utilized with the individual and collective level of consciousness we had reached. Finally, drawing from my own life experiences, encounters, observations of different people and situations, how religion and spirituality could be related to medicine, to healthcare and wellbeing, at a time when the medical paradigm is shifting and changing, both quantitatively and qualitatively speaking, and when "higher help" is desperately needed not only to "live well" but also to survive at this critical historical juncture of our evolution.

To this end, I dedicated the first part of this work (originally, its first volume) to *religion*, by focusing upon and seeking to provide a short but meaningful synopsis of the seven great world religions: the four Eastern (Hinduism, Confucianism, Taoism, and Buddhism) and the three Western religions (Judaism, Christianity, and Islam). This could obviously be an immense and unfinished task, and so I decided to take Huston Smith's, The *Religions of Man*, as my basic and direct "model" and "point of reference", and attempt a brief and concise summary of each that would aim at highlighting its basic fundamentals. The larger perspective into which I embedded this endeavor was the spiritual tradition my own personal experiences. Here I tried to describe and suggest why religion has always been so important to human beings and what it might provide to them to realize their most important needs and aspirations.

The second part of this work (originally its second volume) focused upon *spirituality*, which is the true "end" of all authentic religion, by focusing upon and attempting to provide a rational theoretical framework to present its basic nature, distinctive features, dynamics, manifestations, and contributions. Here I was also inspired by Huston's Smith's *Forgotten Truth: The Primordial Tradition* but in a more indirect way. My essential "reference points" and models here were, again, the spiritual tradition, the Eastern Orthodox Church, and psychosynthesis, all of which blended into and were interpreted through my own personal experiences and level of consciousness and being. In a sense this was easier than for the first part as the materials are less complex and diversified but also more profound as genuine spirituality can only be rooted in direct personal experience . . . for which we do not yet have an adequate vocabulary!

It is for this reason (because we lack appropriate concepts, because spirituality is relatively "new" or restricted to few people and thus not part of the dominant culture, and because it is quite "personal" with a multitude of facets pointing to the same reality) that I have deliberately been "repetitive", "redundant", and somewhat "pedantic" in repeating and looking at the same thing over and over again but from *different angles*! Forty years of university teaching, in different languages, countries, and subjects have taught me that this is a very important pedagogical instrument that will go a long way to make people understand better what is being said and presented to be able to remember it and integrate it with the body of their cognitive knowledge. Thus this was done *deliberately* on my part and I hope you will forgive me for its apparent meticulousness and "redundancy".

The third part (originally the third volume) of this work was designed to apply the core perspective, theory, assumptions, insights, and ideas of religion and spirituality to medicine, healthcare and wellness; this for several reasons all of which are quite important. First, we are now living at a truly critical time, perhaps the most crucial passage and transformation in human evolution, when human consciousness is definitely expanding and entering into a higher level or "floor" of the inner sky-scraper (specifically when we are moving from the 3rd to the 4th and 5th levels).

This *metanoia* also involves major paradigm shifts in all academic fields and professions, notably in the medical field. From a vision of human nature as one-dimensional structure (*homo simplex*) we are now moving on to a multidimensional structure (*homo duplex* and *triplex*) wherein the vitality, the emotions, and the thoughts of a person will play an increasingly more important role. Not only, because of a number of complex internal, external and evolutionary factors, we will no longer be able to "make it" in the 21st century without higher laws, principles, energies and frequencies, which are spiritual in nature and origin. Thus, the traditional "black box" of science composed of our senses, reason and imagination, are no longer adequate to enable us to understand ourselves, the world we live in and the present challenges, dangers and opportunities. Thus spirituality from being and *option* is now becoming a *necessity*. For, indeed, the 21st century will either be spiritual or . . . will not be!

Second, on our path of involution, or descent from spirit into matter, we moved from unity, connectedness, and synthesis, the Great Chain of Being, to multiplicity, separation, and analysis, the fragmented, alienated, and confused modern man! This led us into two "dead-ends": first analyzing the parts at deeper and deeper levels but without taking into account their *relationship to the whole* which is always greater than the sum of its parts. This created a reductionistic and falsified picture of reality . . . which is not longer effective and "alive". Secondly, we also focused on matter and forgot Life which does not come from matter but from elsewhere and thus further alienated ourselves from reality. Religion, the multiple means, and spirituality, the end, now must be reintegrated into science in general and medicine in particular to bring into prominence, connectedness, relationships, and synthesis—LOVE—to balance knowledge and power. Thirdly, we got lost with a great deal of ever-multiplying *details* which, however, leave what is *essential out*, thus creating confusion, dysfunction and pathology.

Thus, the great challenge today is to go back to what is *really essential*, to what makes sense and provides meaning, purpose and value which, in turn will bring hope for the mind, motivation for the heart, and life for the will. To do this we need a new theoretical framework, or "global perspective", which is precisely what religion and spirituality (properly understood and lived) will contribute. Having shown what religion and spirituality are, at least to the extent that this is possible at the present level of consciousness and being, we can now schematize and summarize what their integration in our overall cognitive body of knowledge, in general, and to the medical and healthcare field, in particular, will make possible and what their distinctive contributions might be. Basically, these are:

1. It will make possible as better relationship with and understanding of Reality, both *internal* in the microcosm and at the subjective level, and *external*, in the macrocosm and at the objective level. This by focusing on what is natural, whole, simple, moral, inexpensive, non-dangerous, and more effective.

2. It will offer an integrated perspective where various sectors of the human condition (academic disciplines and professions) can, once again, be connected and seen in a larger interacting whole. Thus, where religion, science, philosophy, education, and healthcare will all be interrelated and interacting with each other.

3. Here the *specialist* will again have to become the *generalist:* by raising our level of consciousness and being it will become more and more important to make "connections", "set up relationships", and "create associations" with a living, dynamic, multidimensional whole. Seen through the perspective, the healthcare specialist will have to be able to act not only as a doctor and a therapist, but also as an educator, a philosopher, an advocate and a trusted friend—as a Sage!

4. Another fundamental point will be the recognition that human beings and thus both doctors and patients are "magnets" and attract both persons and circumstances to themselves and thus also health or illnesses. Healthcare professionals will have to recognize and have the humility to accept that they cannot work with and heal "everybody"; that there are certain types of persons and certain specific persons with whom they were meant to work and with whom they can achieve the best results, taking the "destiny" of each into consideration.

5. Professions will to once again become "vocations" (as they once were); namely something you do because you feel that this is what you came in this world to do (to actualize your own potentials and be of service to others) and not something that you do "for making a living", earning some money and obtaining a social position and status! Healthcare, religion, and education would certainly fall in this category!

6. Most important, it will have to realize and act upon the fact that human nature, the universe and life and thus health, illness and healing, just like knowledge or any other fundamental pursuit, always contain a spiritual, a human and a physical dimension which must be integrated and recognized . . . if we want to be connected to Reality, inner and outer, and be effective in what we do.

7. It will have to recognize and accept the fact that we come in this world for a purpose and not by "chance or hazard" thus that we all have a "destiny" and a "duty" to accomplish here that our own higher Self has chosen even before we were born. That being able to fulfill that duty and destiny is, in itself, a most powerful "medicine" and "therapy" to re-harmonize ourselves, detoxify from the various poisons we have set in motion, and to reconnect with our Source.

8. Lastly, it will have to recognize and act on the fact that our true "life and home" are not in this perishable world of duality which is inexorably subject to entropy or decay but in higher dimensional worlds whence we came and wither we are going. In other words, that here we can only pursue that which is *temporal* in nature and which, therefore, can never, fully and completely, fulfill and satisfy us . . . for our higher Self knows and longs for that which is *eternal*, infinite and whole.

To put it into a nutshell: The perspective and paradigm that are emerging on the horizon will very clearly point out that *love* is the truly essential quality of human nature and the human condition and that, as such, it should assume pre-eminence and priority in our lives. And to "love" means to be able to establish a "right and alive relationship" so that we can make exchanges and mutually enrich each other. This is why the world of duality and the "other" was created . . . so that love may manifest, grow, and flourish. Seen in this perspective, integral health will place a great deal of emphasis upon being happy and appreciating what we are living through; upon understanding and being able to be "true to one's self" and to do our "duty" and thus fulfill our destiny in this world. It will mean growing, maturing, and expanding our consciousness and encountering new emergent and dynamic levels wherein the extraordinary adventure and journey of Life can manifest themselves.

What we are witnessing and living through today is a major expansion and transformation of consciousness with new and higher energies, laws and faculties being activated that demand major transformations and readjustments . . . that can be quite complex, confusing and painful! We are moving from the 3rd to the 4th and even the 5th level of consciousness and being where each major passage demands and entails a "death" and "resurrection", a letting go of an older identity and form (or organization) to enter into new and different ones where new needs, aspirations, and parameters will apply. In a sense it is really like having to "face the unknown" (which is terrifying . . . at least for some) in order to discover through direct and personal experience that this "unknown" is orderly, is wise, and is good; hence, that the whole journey, however difficult, painful and confusing, was really more than worth it.

At this new level and once we enter into the 5th level, in a serious and objective way, we will at long last discover that it is possible to "bring all the pieces together", that it is possible to integrate and reconcile all paradoxes and contradictions, "to find true justice, meaning, and purpose" in life and thus to "accept the unacceptable", to "understand the non-intelligible" . . . and to find ourselves, our true and Greater Self as well as God or the Creator of both ourselves, the universe, and Life. That is what I see ahead of us and that is what I would define as the Great Challenge of our times . . . but, in ultimate analysis, it is only something that each and every individual must realize and achieve for himself/herself . . . with the help of divine guidance! And it is to this end, to complete the Great Work together, that I have written this and all the other books I have authored, taught all the classes and seminars in the last 40 years, and lived through all the "crazy" experiences and adventures that were part of my destiny. I sincerely believe that if you do the work required, you all also come to the same conclusion . . . and then truly LIVE and REJOICE!

Bibliography

The importance of bibliography is *relative* depending on who is reading a given book and for what purpose. Scholars, students of a given field, and intellectuals will find an extensive bibliography quite important. Mystics and practical persons, on the other hand, will find it much less important. If there is a only a "rough vocabulary" and few legitimate sources that are available or if a person is more interested in the core materials presented and the personal experience these materials point to, a bibliography is less or even not important. In the past, I have swung from one end of the pendulum to the other by either providing an extensive bibliography or skipping it altogether. For the present work and in view of its fundamental importance, I have decided to find a "golden mean" between these two extremes. At the beginning of this work I have provided a list of my most important works in the three languages that I write and work in and, at the end, a selected biography of the most important authors and works that can significantly contribute to delving deeper into our subject matter.

Assagioli, Roberto. *Psychosynthesis: A Manual of Principles and Techniques*, Viking Viking Press, 1965.
The Act of Will, Viking Press, 1973.
Le Vie dello Spirito (Considerator), Guiseppe Filipponio, 1971.

Bedrij, Orest.   *Celebrate your Divinity*, Xlibris, 2005.
Seeing God Face to Face, Xlibris, 2005.

Bertholet, Dr. Edouard. *La Réincarnation d'après Maître Philippe de Lyons*, Editions Rosicruiciennes, 1864.
Les Mystères de la Grande Tradition Rosicrucienne, idem, 1965.
La Réincarnation, idem, 1965.

Boucher, Laurent.   *Brother André: The Miracle Man of Mount Royal*, St. Joseph Oratory, 1997.

Bucke, Richard.   *Cosmic Consciousness*, Dutton & Co., 1969.

Conforto, Gaetano.   *La Medicina della Luce*, Macro Edizioni, 1004.

Dossey, Larry.   *Recovering the Soul*, Harper, 1089.
                      Reinventing Medicine, idem, 1999.
                      Prayer is good Medicine, idem, 2000.

Eckarstheusen, Karl von. *The Cloud upon the Sanctuary*, SRIA, 1952.

Eliade, Mircea.   *The Sacred and the Profane*, Harper Torchbook, 1959.
                      Myth, Dreams, and Mysteries, idem, 1957.
                      The Two and the One, idem, 1962.

Encause, Dr. Philippe. *Le Maître Philippe de Lyons*, Villain et Belhomme, 1974.

Fontaine, Dr. Janine. *La Médecine du Corps Energétique,* Robert Laffont, 1983.
                      Médecins des trois Corps, idem, 1980.
                      Nos trois Corps et les trois Mondes, idem, 1986.

Fortune, Dion.   *The Work and Training of an Initiate*, Weiser, 1976.
                      The Esoteric Orders and their Work, idem, 1973.
                      The Mystical Quabalah, idem, 1973.

Giovetti, Paula. *Roberto Assagioli: la vita e l'opera del fondatore della psicosintesi*,
                      Edizioni Mediterranee, 1995.

Groening, Bruno, Grete Hausler. *Here is the Truth about Bruno Groening*, Grete
                      Hausler
                      GmbH Verlag, 2002.
                      Matthias Kamp. *A Revolution in Medicine*, idem, 2000.
                      Thomas Busse. *The Miracle Healings of Bruno Groening*,
                      idem, 2004.
                      Kurt Trampler. *The Great Turning Point*, idem, 2002.

James, William. *The Variety of Religious Experience*, Modern Library, 1962.

Keyes, Ken. *Handbook to Higher Consciousness*, Living Love Center, 1074.

Knight, Gareth.   *Experience of the inner Worlds*, Helios Book, 1975.
                      A Practical Guide to Quabalistic Symbolism, idem, 1965.

Lebrun, Maguy.   *Médecins du Ciel, Médecins de la Terre*, Robert Laffont, 1987.
L'Amour en Partage, idem, 1991.
La Joie qui soulève les Montagnes, idem, 1999.

Loski, Vladimir.   *The Mystical Theology of the Eastern Church*, James Clarke, 1957.

Markides, Kyriacos.   *Gifts of the Desert: The Forgotten Path of Christian Spirituality*, Doubleday, 2005.
The Mountain of Silence, Doubleday Anchor, 2001.
Fire in the Heart: Healers, Sages and Mystics, Routledge & Kegan Paul, 1990.

Maslow, Abraham.   *Towards a Psychology of Being*, Van Nostrand, 1971.
The Farther Reaches of Human Nature, Viking Press, 1971.

Mouni Sadhu.   *Concentration*, Wilshire Books, 1973.
Meditation, George Allen & Unwin, 1969.
Theurgy, idem, 1965.

Mouravieff, Boris.   *Gnosis: Studies and Commentaries on the Esoteric Tradition of Eastern Orthodoxy*, Praxis Institute Press, 1990.

Papus. *L'Occultisme*, Robert Laffont, 1975.

Pavese, Armando. *Guarigioni Miracolose in tutte le Religioni*, Piemme, 2005.

Plummer, George. *Rosicrucian Fundamentals*, SRIA, 1920.

Saint Denis, Jean de. *Technique de la Prière*, Présence Orthodoxe, 1971.
Initiation a la Genèse, idem, 1971.

Sédir, Paul.   *Initiations*, Bibliothèque des Amitiés Spirituelles, 1956.
La Prière, idem, 1956.
La Guérison du Christ, idem, 1953.

Smith, Huston.   *The Religions of Man*, Harper & Row, 1956.
Forgotten Truth: The Primordial Tradition, idem, 1976.
The Soul of Christianity, Harper Collins, 2002.
The Way Things Are, University of California, 2005.

Underhill, Evelyn. *Mysticism*, E.R. Dutton, 1919.
Worship, Harper & Brothers, 1937.
Practical Mysticism, E.P. Dutton, 1943.

Vigorelli, Piero. *Miracoli: Guarigioni, Prodigi e Apparizioni in Italia e nel Mondo*, Piemme, 2002.
Nuovi Miracoli e Guarigioni Straordinarie, idem, 2003.

Zamperini, Roberto. *Energie Sottili e la Terapia Energo-Vibrazionale*, Macro Edizioni, 2002.